Medicine

✚⇒ Topics and Problems

EMERGENCY
Medicine

✚⇨ Topics and Problems

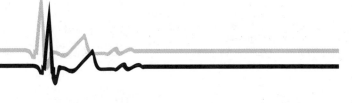

Prof George Jelinek MD Dip DHM FACEM
Professor and Chairman of Emergency Medicine

Dr Ian Rogers MBBS FACEM
Director of Emergency Medicine

Sir Charles Gairdner Hospital
Perth, Australia

b

**Blackwell
Science
Asia**

©1999 by Blackwell Science Asia Pty Ltd

Published by Blackwell Science Asia Pty Ltd

First printed 1999

Editorial Offices:

54 University Street, Carlton South,
Victoria 3053, Australia
Osney Mead. Oxford OX2 OEL, UK
25 John Street, London WC IN 2BL, UK
23 Ainslie Place, Edinburgh EH3 6AJ, UK
350 Main Street, Malden,
MA 02148-5018, USA

Other Editorial Offices:

Blackwell Wissenschafts-Verlag GmbH
Kurfilrstendamm 57
10707 Berlin, Germany
Zehemergasse 6
1140 Wien, Austria

Designed by Tom Kurema
Typeset by J&M Typesetting
Edited by Scharlaine Cairns,
Charlie C. Editorial Pty Ltd.
Printed in Australia

DISTRIBUTORS

Blackwell Science Pty Ltd
54 University Street,
Carlton South, Victoria 3053, Australia

Orders Tel: 03 9347 0300
Fax: 03 9349 3016
E-mail: info@blacksci-asia.com.au
Internet: www.blackwell-science-asia.com.au

North-America

Blackwell Science, Inc.
Commerce Place, 350 Main Street
Malden. MA 02148-5018

Orders Tel: 617388 8250
              800759 6102
Fax: 617388 8255

Canada

Copp Clark Professional
200 Adelaide Street, West, 3rd Floor,
Toronto, Ontario M5H IW7

Orders Tel: 416597 1616
              800 8159417
Fax: 416597 1616

United Kingdom

Marston Book Services Ltd
PO Box 87
Oxford, OX2 ODT

Orders Tel: 01865 791155
Fax: 01865 791927
Telex: 837515

Cataloguing-in-Publication Data

Jelinek. George A.
Emergency medicine: topics and problems

ISBN 0 86793 013 6.

1. Emergency medicine. I. Rogers, Ian, 1961-.
II. Title.

616.025

Foreword

To many of us, emergency medicine is the most interesting and stimulating branch of medicine. It has made huge strides forward in the past 20 years. After the American College of Emergency Physicians was formed 25 years ago, many other countries took up the torch. In no country has this field been more eagerly welcomed than in Australia. Those of us who have watched that development regard it as a great privilege to have done so.

In the 1950s, there was no formal training in emergency medicine at undergraduate or postgraduate level. Little changed in the 20 years that followed, although the Platt report in the UK (1962) recognised that some reorganisation was needed. However, medicine itself was changing as society changed. There was improved technology, and increasing specialisation often because of the technology. Antibiotics arrived in the 1940s and, suddenly, fatal illnesses became almost incidental. The average age of the population rose rapidly, for no longer was the 'old people's friend' (pneumonia) the end of the road. Anaesthetics, surgery, and many other fields developed with breathtaking speed. Intensive care was born from the advent of ventilation technology. Unfortunately, disease did not stand still either. Many illnesses that are now household words were unknown in 1952 when I qualified. Cigarette smoking was just becoming to be recognised for the lethal addiction that it is. Acute myocardial infarction, also very largely smoking related, became common. As cars proliferated, the road trauma epidemic developed.

One of the most significant developments arising from these changes was that middle class patients started being taken to public hospitals. The poor had always relied on public hospitals and the rich had other avenues of help. The middle class had always called their own doctors. But road crashes require immediate attention and ambulance transport to take the injured to hospital. In the same way, heart attacks require urgent help.

The miracle of defibrillation, with the resuscitation skills of expired air ventilation and external cardiac compression, made it possible for the first time to save patients after cardiac arrest. These factors combined to thrust the emergency department into the limelight. The first television emergency department show, *Emergency Ward Ten*, was shown in the UK in the early 1960s.

In Australia, although these changes were occurring, nothing happened in the medical field until the end of the 1960s, when the first 'casualty supervisors' were appointed. Progress since then has been spectacular, with the formation of the Australasian College for Emergency Medicine in 1983, the development of the Australasian journal *Emergency Medicine* from 1989, and the recognition of emergency medicine as a principal speciality in 1993. Whether it was welcomed or not, emergency medicine arrived with a bang, to be thrust onto the centre of the medical stage.

The undergraduate curriculum has been slow to reflect this progress. Until very recently, medical students have had less experience and much less instruction in emergency medicine than they did 40 years ago. Then they had three or four weeks of experience in the old 'casualty department', even if there was no formal instruction. Thanks to the 'sister in charge', helped by the occasional registrar, there was practical help and instruction by the bedside. The Australian Medical Council has now insisted that medical students receive teaching in practical procedures and in the management of emergencies. Gradually the universities are making time in the curriculum for this, despite the competing demands of every other specialist discipline.

At last there will be a generation of doctors who understand the basic principles of emergency care. So now, at long last, here is a text book written to help medical students do exactly that. The authors are both distinguished in teaching as well as in emergency medicine. George Jelinek is the first full Professor of Emergency Medicine in Australasia, and has played a very large part in the establishment of one of the most successful training schools for emergency physicians. Ian Rogers has been part of a team in Melbourne which has been well known for postgraduate training and he has been Senior Lecturer in Auckland for two years, where he started the first course for medical students in emergency medicine. Both authors have had extensive experience of teaching undergraduates, and their joint enthusiasm is highly infectious.

The authors have arranged the book in two parts. The first and longest part gives short accounts of many of the most important emergency problems. The other part comprises a number of clinical problems aimed at giving a 'real life' insight into what may happen and what the skilled helper can do. Any student who has read through this book with care (for it is very concentrated information) will be far better equipped to help an emergency patient than before.

I wish I'd had such a book when I was a student—but it would have been a very much slimmer volume, because the larger part of it could not have been written then. As today's authors write, the winners will be the millions of patients who attend our Australasian hospital emergency departments every year. This book will do much to ensure that they continue to be winners.

Edward Brentnall
Emeritus Consultant in Emergency Medicine
Box Hill Hospital, Victoria

Contents

Preface

The Australian Medical Council has found that medical students are graduating from medical school without the necessary knowledge and skills to manage common emergencies. This book is our attempt to redress the balance a little, by providing simple clinical guidelines and information about the common medical problems and situations students may encounter in their hospital attachments. The topics are not intended to be exhaustive, nor is the book intended to be a comprehensive reference book. We have chosen a somewhat eclectic list of topics that reflects our particular interests—however we feel that they largely represent the core of the unique body of knowledge that is emergency medicine, with information distilled from extensive clinical experience and reading of the literature. Our hope is that there is not only enough information to enable the student intern to manage common emergencies, but that the practical tips and advice provided will help students acquire the necessary skills easily and quickly.

Part 2, comprising clinical problems, is included because we recognise that problem-based learning results in better retention of information. Working through these cases with classmates and clinical teachers will, we hope, better prepare students for the inevitable day when they must manage such cases themselves.

The preparation of a textbook inevitably reduces the time available to spend with family. We thank our families for their patience and understanding in this process. We also thank Janet Carr for her secretarial support and continuing attention to detail. Our sincere thanks must go to our emergency physician colleagues in Auckland and Perth whose advice and cooperation has been invaluable.

Finally we thank the University of Western Australia and the Sir Charles Gairdner Hospital for establishing the first bona fide academic emergency medicine unit in Australia. This recognition of the fundamental importance of teaching emergency medicine to students should be the catalyst for other medical schools around our region to follow suit, and accord emergency medicine the place in academic medicine it deserves. The beneficiaries, after all, will be the millions of patients who are forced to attend Australasian emergency departments every year due to unforeseen sudden illness or injury.

George Jelinek
and **Ian Rogers**

EMERGENCY MEDICINE TOPICS

GUIDELINES FOR CARDIOPULMONARY RESUSCITATION/ ADVANCED CARDIAC LIFE SUPPORT

A number of organisations publish guidelines and algorithms for the management of cardiorespiratory arrest. The most comprehensive are those produced by the American Heart Association, last published in *JAMA* in October 1992*, and due to be updated in the year 2000. Perhaps the easiest to understand, though, are those produced by the Australian Resuscitation Council, a copy of which, with modifications, is reproduced in flow chart form as Figure 1 on the following page. During your student years you should receive more extensive advanced cardiac life support (ACLS) training.

Although the algorithms may look complex, it is important to emphasise that results in cardiopulmonary resuscitation (CPR) are usually produced by:

- airway management
- early defibrillation
- adrenaline.

The therapies further along the algorithms than these are, at best, of limited value. Rather than trying to memorise the whole algorithm, be sure that you understand the basic and initial steps first. These are the therapies that usually save lives.

---

* 'Guidelines for cardiopulmonary resuscitation and emergency cardiac care', Emergency Cardiac Care Committee and Subcommittees, American Heart Association, *JAMA*, October 28, 1992.

CARDIAC ARREST

▼ Advanced life support flowchart†

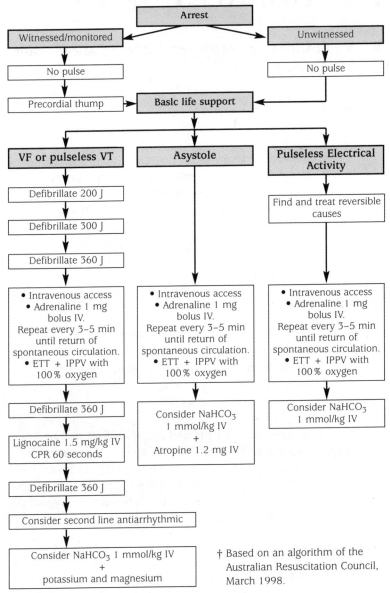

Figure 1

ARREST DRUG RATIONALES

▼ **Medications potentially useful in advanced adult life support**

Adrenaline

Action

Adrenaline is a naturally occurring catecholamine with α and β effects. The α-adrenergic action is important in cardiac arrest as it produces peripheral vasoconstriction and directs available cardiac output to the myocardium and brain. Adrenaline facilitates defibrillation by improving myocardial blood flow during cardio-pulmonary resuscitation (CPR). It is the most important drug in advanced life support.

Indications

- Ventricular fibrillation after initial counter shocks have failed.
- Initial treatment of asystole and pulseless electrical activity.

Dose

The initial adult dose is 1 mg and this should be repeated at regular intervals (every 3–5 min) during CPR. Further bolus doses or continuous infusion may be required to maintain an adequate blood pressure after the patient-generated pulse has returned. If an infusion is necessary, it should be delivered via a dedicated central line as soon as possible.

Complications

- Tachyarrhythmias due to β_1 effects.
- Severe hypertension after resuscitation.

- Tissue necrosis if extravasation occurs.
- Inactivation of adrenaline if mixed with sodium bicarbonate.

Lignocaine

Action

Lignocaine is a potent suppressor of abnormal cardiac excitability.

Indications

- Antiarrhythmic of first choice for ventricular fibrillation (VF) and ventricular tachycardia (VT).
- Multiple DC shocks and adrenaline have failed to revert VF.
- Prophylaxis for recurrent VF or VT.

Dose

Initial dose is 1.5 mg/kg. During resuscitation an additional bolus dose of 0.5 mg/kg may be considered.

Complications

- Neurological — drowsiness, agitation, twitching, fits and coma.
- Cardiac — hypotension, bradycardia, heart block and asystole.

Bretylium

Action

Bretylium lowers the defibrillation threshold and restores the fibrillation threshold to normal.

Indications

- Second line antiarrhythmic for VF and VT.
- After defibrillation, adrenaline and lignocaine have failed to revert VF.
- If VF has recurred despite the use of lignocaine.
- If other measures have failed to revert VT.

Dose

Initial bolus of 5mg/kg. A subsequent dose of 10 mg/kg can be given after five minutes.

Note

This drug was discontinued by the sole manufacturer in Australasia in May 1997.

Complications

There is potential for hypotension.

Atropine

Action

This parasympathetic blocker antagonises the action of the vagus nerve on the heart.

Indications

- In bradyarrhythmia to increase the heart rate.
- When asystole is resistant to standard treatment.

Dose

It is given as a bolus of 1.2 mg in asystole or as 0.6 mg increments in bradycardia, to a maximum of 2.4 mg.

Complications

- Cardiac — tachycardia, which may cause hypotension.

- Neurological — excitement, delirium.
- Hyperthermia (in large doses).

Potassium

Action

Potassium is an electrolyte essential for membrane stability. A low serum potassium level, especially in conjunction with digoxin therapy and hypomagnesaemia, leads to life threatening ventricular arrhythmias.

Indications

- Persistent VF in patients who have taken diuretics without potassium supplementation.
- Documented hypokalaemia.

Dose

A bolus of 2.5 mmol is given intravenously.

Complications

- Inappropriate or excessive use will produce hyperkalaemia with bradycardia, hypotension and possible asystole.
- Extravasation may lead to tissue necrosis.

Magnesium

Action

Magnesium is an essential electrolyte. Low serum magnesium may be caused by diuretic use, severe diarrhoea and alcohol abuse. Hypomagnesaemia causes myocardial hyper-excitability particularly in the presence of hypokalaemia and digoxin therapy.

Indications

- Torsades de pointes.
- Arrhythmias associated with digoxin toxicity.
- Ventricular arrhythmias.
- Documented hypokalaemia.

Dose

It is given as a 5 mmol bolus of magnesium sulfate, which may be repeated once followed by an infusion of 20 mmol over four hours.

Complications

Excessive use may lead to muscle weakness, paralysis and respiratory failure.

Sodium bicarbonate

Action

Sodium bicarbonate is an alkalinising solution which combines with hydrogen ions to produce CO_2 and H_2O. Theoretically it reverses the metabolic acidosis associated with tissue hypoxia in cardiac arrest. In most cardiac arrests, early efficient CPR and adequate ventilation negate the need for any $NaHCO_3$.

Indications

- Treatment of documented metabolic acidosis.
- Hyperkalaemia.
- Protracted cardiac arrest (greater than 15 minutes).

Dose

It is initially given as a bolus of 1 mmol/kg then as guided by arterial blood gas levels. Administration must be accompanied by adequate ventilation and CPR.

Complications

$NaHCO_3$ is no longer routine initial therapy because of the risk of alkalosis, hypernatraemia and hyperosmolarity. Theoretically, cellular acidosis may develop when CO_2, which freely enters the cells, is liberated from HCO_3.

Calcium

Action

This electrolyte is essential for normal muscle and nerve activity. It transiently increases myocardial excitability and contractility and peripheral resistance.

Indications

Calcium is seldom indicated for the management of cardiac arrest. It may be useful in the treatment of arrhythmias or hypotension associated with hyperkalaemia, hypocalcaemia or overdose of calcium-channel blocking drugs.

Dose

The usual adult bolus dose is 5–10 mL of 10% calcium chloride.

Complications

- It may increase myocardial and cerebral injury by mediating cell death.
- Extravasation produces tissue necrosis.

CARDIAC AND RESPIRATORY ARREST IN CHILDREN

Cardiac arrest in children, unlike arrest in adults, is not usually a primary event, but is secondary to respiratory obstruction or failure. Priorities in cardiac arrest in children are given below.

(i)   Restore ventilation
- Clear the airway of any foreign material and maintain patency using a:
  - backward head tilt (except in trauma)
  - chin lift
  - jaw thrust.
- Begin artificial ventilation using 100% oxygen by bag and mask. If unavailable, use expired air resuscitation.
- If a clear airway cannot be obtained, intubate.
- Endotracheal tube (ETT) size is 'age divided by 4 plus 4', uncuffed under 8 years of age.
- Try to avoid gastric distension.

(ii)   Restore circulation
- Start external cardiac compression (ECC) without delay and maintain if cardiac arrest is confirmed (by unconsciousness, absent pulses or cardiac impulse, absent respiration and dilated pupils).
- Use two fingers for infants, or the heel of the hand for children aged 1–8 years.
- Continue external cardiac massage without pauses for ventilation (when there are two resuscitators).
- The resuscitator giving ventilation should time the ventilations between massage compressions so that there is no pause between compressions.
- The rates per minute for one and two person resuscitation are in the table on the next page.

		Neonate	Child/infant	Adult
One person	Ventilation	16	12	8
	Compression	120	90	60
Two person	Ventilation	24–30	20	12
	Compression	120–150	100	60

(iii) **Obtain vascular access**
- Insert an intravenous (IV) line into a hand or arm vein.
- Give all drugs by this route.
- If peripheral vascular access is difficult, don't delay in using other routes.

(iv) **Alternative routes**
- Other veins (external jugular, leg, femoral, neck, scalp in infants).
- Intraosseous (IO): using a commercial intraosseous needle, try proximal and distal tibia, and the iliac crest. Drugs and IV fluids can be given IO.
- Endotracheal: adrenaline, lignocaine and atropine can be given. Drug doses should be larger than for intravenous use (up to 10 times), diluted with normal saline (newborns 1 mL, up to 5 mL for school-age children), and given via a catheter down the tube. Bicarbonate and calcium are not recommended by this route.

(v) **Defibrillate/monitor ECG**
- Attach electro-cardiograph (ECG) leads as soon as possible.
- For ventricular fibrillation or ventricular tachycardia, use 4–5 joules/kg DC countershock. Use paediatric paddles up to one year of age.

(vi) **Use drugs as appropriate**
- Adrenaline: the initial dose is 0.01 mg/kg. Usually no other drugs are used. Increase the dose to a maximum 0.2 mg/kg if no response.

- Sodium bicarbonate: the value is debatable. Initial dose is 2 mmol/kg followed by 1 mmol/kg every 10 minutes until effective ventilation and cardiac output are restored .

FAILED AIRWAY MANAGEMENT

▼ Clinical features

Failure to gain control of a patient's airway may occur because of operator inexperience, the anatomy of the patient's airway (bullneck or receding jaw), the view being obscured by blood or vomit, or airway distortion (such as with trauma or epiglottitis).

Although definitive airway control is always the ultimate aim, patients die initially of hypoxaemia and hypercarbia. Oxygenation (and ventilation) is always the highest priority and the prime concern in failed airway protocols.

▼ Management

A suggested algorithm is shown in Figure 2 on the next page.

Useful tools in airway management

Introducer

The conventional coated wire introducer is lubricated and put inside an endotracheal tube with the end still concealed in the end of the tube. It is bent into a 'hockey stick' shape, so that it guides the tip of the tube to an anteriorly placed larynx. If time permits, this should be used as a routine part of all emergency intubations.

Bougie

The flexible bougie is used in a similar shape to the coated wire introducer but the bougie protrudes from the tube and the tube is advanced over it. The aim is to place the tip of the bougie at or just through the vocal cords.

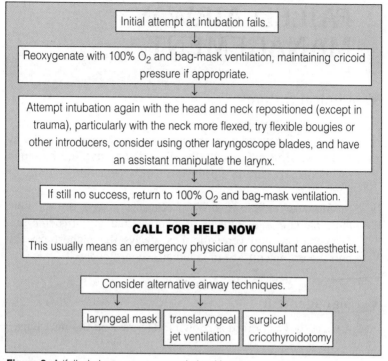

Figure 2: A 'failed airway management' algorithm.

Laryngeal mask

The laryngeal mask is lubricated and introduced with its concavity anteriorly, with the patient's head positioned in the usual airway position. A laryngoscope is not used. The mask is advanced until a definite resistance is felt and then the cuff is inflated with 30 mL or so of air. A size 6.0 endotracheal tube can often be passed through the laryngeal mask and will come to lie in the larynx.

Translaryngeal jet ventilation

Translaryngeal jet ventilation requires a specific jet ventilation device which runs directly from a wall oxygen source and not through a conventional oxygen flow meter. The jet ventilator is connected to a 14G IV catheter that has been passed through the cricothyroid membrane.

Surgical cricothyroidotomy

To perform a surgical cricothyroidotomy:

- fully extend the neck
- make a vertical, midline 2.5 cm incision centred over the cricothyroid membrane
- pull the margins of the incision laterally to make it lie transverse
- stab a hole through the membrane
- if necessary, enlarge the hole with the handle of the scalpel
- insert a size 6.0 endotracheal tube and inflate the cuff.

SEVERE ASTHMA

▼ Clinical features

Asthma can be acutely graded into mild, moderate and severe on the basis of clinical presentation using peak expiratory flow rate (PEFR), speech patterns, SaO_2 readings and mental state as indicators.

Grade	PEFR	Speech	SaO2	Mental state
Mild	> 75% predicted	sentences	normal	normal
Moderate	25–75% predicted	phrases	↓(90–94%)	normal
Severe	< 25% predicted	words or nil	↓↓ (< 90%)	depressed

Arterial blood gases (ABGs) are only infrequently performed. If done in the mild case, they will show a respiratory alkalosis. Normal pH and pCO_2 in the patient with clinically moderate or severe asthma is an ominous sign of potential respiratory failure. ABGs should be reserved for the severe case. Consider a chest X-ray only in the non-responsive severe case and in any case where there is a rapid decline despite treatment. Look for complications such as pneumothorax, pneumomediastinum, infection, arrhythmias, theophylline toxicity and hypokalaemia.

▼ Management

In the severe case treatment includes:

- high flow O_2
- continuous nebulised salbutamol (5 mg in 3 mL saline)
- nebulised ipratropium (0.5 mg stat and four hourly)
- hydrocortisone (200 mg IV), or dexamethasone (8 mg IV) or prednisolone (50 mg per oral)
- considering salbutamol (250 mg IV and infusion) or adrenaline (infusion or subcutaneous/intramuscular).

Optional treatment in severe cases includes Mg^{2+}, ketamine, halothane, heliox, glucagon and IV aminophylline, none of which has been shown conclusively to have benefit.

Patients with mild asthma can usually be discharged. All patients with severe asthma should be admitted at least overnight, even if they respond rapidly to treatment. They may need intensive care unit attention.

Assisted expiration may be of benefit in the most severe cases with gas trapping. Intubation and ventilation should generally be considered as a last resort, but should not be withheld until after arrest in the rapidly deteriorating asthmatic.

PULMONARY OEDEMA

▼ Clinical features

Pulmonary oedema can manifest in varying degrees of severity. The classic patient with florid pulmonary oedema sits upright, is sweaty and agitated with tachycardia and hypertension, and has obvious crepitations on auscultation.

'Cardiac asthma' is a real clinical entity, though rare. Such patients present with bronchospasm alone but either treatment or chest X-ray reveals underlying pulmonary oedema.

▼ Management

A step-by-step management plan for severe pulmonary oedema is:

- sit the patient upright, calm and reassure
- administer high flow O_2 and monitor ECG, blood pressure, SaO_2
- establish IV access (no fluids)
- send bloods for urea and electrolytes, full blood examination, and cardiac enzymes
- metoclopramide (10 mg IV) as an antiemetic if required
- nitrates (depending on blood pressure) given sublingually, as a paste/patch topically, or as an IV infusion (glyceryl trinitrate at 2.5–20 µg/min)
- diuresis with frusemide, 40 mg IV or at least the patient's usual daily dose intravenously (repeat diuretics every 15 minutes as required)
- morphine in 1–2.5 mg IV aliquots as required (it is both anxiolytic and a vasodilator, but avoid large doses which depress respiration and conscious state)
- ECG to exclude underlying infarct or arrhythmia
- chest X-ray to confirm clinical diagnosis of left ventricular failure.

For the most severe or unresponsive cases consider:

- continuous positive airway pressure (CPAP)
- inotropes
- assisted ventilation
- intubation and ventilatory support.

PULMONARY EMBOLISM

▼ Clinical features

Pulmonary embolism (PE) is graded (i) to (v) according to the following classification:

- **(i)** asymptomatic
- **(ii)** symptomatic, haemodynamically stable
- **(iii)** hypotensive responding to fluid loading
- **(iv)** hypotensive requiring vasopressor support
- **(v)** arrested.

Symptoms can be indistinguishable from many other acute respiratory emergencies but include sudden chest pain (90%), dyspnoea (85%), cough (50%), haemoptysis (30%), and collapse (10%). Signs are similarly non-specific and include tachypnoea (90%), tachycardia (45%), fever (45%), hypotension (uncommonly), and signs of deep vein thrombosis (< 30%).

The ECG is abnormal in about 85% of cases but only with tachycardia or non-specific ST/T changes. The classic S_1, Q_3, T_3 pattern of acute right heart strain is present in only 10% of cases. Chest X-ray usually appears abnormal but no changes are specific. It may show atelectasis, elevated diaphragm, oligaemic lung (Westermark's sign) or a wedge-shaped infarct (Hampton's hump). Only 7–22% of cases are normal. Arterial blood gases show an increased A-a gradient in 85% of cases.

D-Dimer assay, even if normal, does not exclude PE. Latex tests particularly are not very sensitive. However the newer 'Simpli-Red' test may be sensitive enough to use to exclude the disease.

Ventilation perfusion (V/Q) scans may be helpful but are often non-contributory.

- Low V/Q probability   PE likelihood 15%
- Intermediate V/Q probability   PE likelihood 30%
- High V/Q probability   PE likelihood 90%

The V/Q scan probability must be assessed in the light of the clinical probability.

▼ Management

- Grades (i), (ii), (iii): oxygen, heparin 5000 units stat then 1000 units/hour
- Grades (iii), (iv), (v): oxygen, streptokinase 250 000 units over 10 minutes then 100 000 units/hour, volume replacement and vasopressors. An alternative to streptokinase is r-PA, particularly when the patient is in extremis, because the drug is given more rapidly as bolus injections.

BARTS & THE LONDON QMSMD

PNEUMOTHORAX

▼ **Clinical features**

Pneumothorax may be spontaneous or traumatic. Traumatic pneumothorax occurs usually in the setting of multi-trauma but can be iatrogenic. It may be due to attempts at central venous catheterisation and various interventional radiological procedures.

▼ **Management**

Conservative management

Small minimally symptomatic pneumothoraces (< 20%) can be managed by observation only on an outpatient basis.

Catheter aspiration

Larger pneumothoraces are managed by catheter aspiration as follows.

- Insert a long 14G or 16G intravenous cannula attached to a 10 mL syringe into the second intercostal space in the mid-clavicular line until air is aspirated. Local anaesthetic is required. Continuous aspiration will confirm correct position. There are now several commercial varieties of catheter which are flexible and will not kink, and have multiple openings near the tip to avoid occlusion during aspiration.
- Advance the catheter further and attach to a 50 mL syringe and three-way tap via a length of extension tubing.
- Aspirate (expelling via the three-way tap) until no more can be aspirated or more than 3000 mL has been taken.

- Perform a repeat chest X-ray.
- If there is a small pneumothorax or no pneumothorax remaining, follow up as an outpatient.
- Observe overnight if there is underlying lung disease such as chronic airflow limitation.
- A larger remaining pneumothorax requires referral for inpatient care and possible chest tube insertion using a small tube (e.g. 16Fr).

Chest tube

- Chest tube insertion. Tension pneumothorax can be managed by needle aspiration in an emergency before proceeding to formal intercostal chest tube.

In general, traumatic pneumothorax is treated with a large bore (32Fr or larger) chest tube inserted through the fifth intercostal space in the mid-axillary line. The large tube is needed for the blood which is likely to drain from a traumatic pneumothorax. The tube should always be inserted using a blunt dissection technique without a trochar. Drainage of greater than 1500 mL of blood initially, or greater than 250 mL per hour subsequently, is considered an indication for thoracotomy. Needle induced traumatic pneumothoraces may be suitable for the catheter aspiration technique outlined above.

MANAGEMENT OF OTHER ARRHYTHMIAS

▼ Ventricular tachycardia

If unstable (blood pressure < 90 mmHg systolic, altered conscious state, chest pain, cardiac failure) with ventricular tachycardia (VT):

- sedate (if required) with low dose midazolam
- use cardioversion using synchronised DC countershock, 100 J.

If stable, treat as follows:

- oxygen
- lignocaine (1–1.5 mg/kg IV bolus)

If no reversion, consider the following treatment:

- sotalol (up to 1.5 mg/kg IV over 10 minutes)
- procainamide (up to 15 mg/kg at no faster than 50 mg/min)
- amiodarone (300 mg over 30 minutes)
- adenosine, 6 mg (+ 12 mg if needed) rapid IV bolus (in case rhythm is supraventricular tachycardia: adenosine will not revert VT)
- correct electrolyte disturbances such as low potassium or magnesium.

If still no reversion, semi-elective cardioversion.

▼ Regular narrow complex tachycardia

If unstable, proceed to sedation and cardioversion with 50–100 J synchronised DC shock.

If stable:

- oxygen
- try vagal manoeuvres (no eyeball pressure) — valsalva manoeuvre with the patient supine is recommended for reasons of safety and efficacy (carotid sinus massage can be tried if this fails – always listen for carotid bruits first).

If no reversion:

- adenosine, 6 mg (+ 12 mg if needed) rapid IV bolus
- consider verapamil 1 mg/min up to 10 mg (watch blood pressure)
- atenolol, as an alternative to verapamil (1 mg/min up to 5 mg).

If no reversion, proceed to sedation and cardioversion.

▼ Atrial fibrillation

- Correct underlying problems such as hypoxaemia, low potassium, cardiac failure.
- Digoxin is the traditional therapy but probably no better than placebo.
- Intravenous calcium channel blockers may offer better rate control but can lead to hypotension due to negative inotropic effects. Sotalol and amiodarone offer small benefits over placebo.

MYOCARDIAL INFARCTION/ THROMBOLYSIS

▼ Clinical features

Acute myocardial infarction (AMI) is a clinical diagnosis. Features include typical crushing, pressing or constricting chest pain or tightness, although many patients with established AMI have atypical pain. The ECG is usually abnormal with localised ST elevation. Q waves indicate full thickness infarction. Patients with normal ECGs who do have AMI have a much lower complication rate.

One-off cardiac enzymes are not helpful in excluding AMI. Serial enzymes over six hours can exclude over 95% of AMIs but, in general, single enzyme results should not guide admission/discharge decisions.

Complications include arrhythmias, cardiac failure and cardiogenic shock.

▼ Management

Treatment of the patient with suspected ischaemic chest pain needs to encompass some or all of the following areas.

- Supportive treatment including oxygen, positioning and reassurance.
- Treat life-threatening problems, principally arrhythmias.
- Monitor ECG, blood pressure and SaO_2.
- Gain IV access. If thrombolysis is planned then two lines are required of at least 18G so that one can be used to give drugs and the other to take blood samples. In the emergency department, K^+ is the

most important test. Group and hold and cardiac
enzymes may be indicated.

- History is only brief and should focus on the
  questions: 'Is this ischaemic chest pain?' and 'Is there
  a need for or contraindication to thrombolysis?'
- The most valuable investigation is the ECG. Compare
  to old ones if available.
- Chest X-ray is not a priority and is really only
  indicated in the emergency department if treatable
  left ventricular failure is suspected.
- The criteria for thrombolysis are constantly evolving
  and depend on a host of factors. The
  contraindications are relative rather than absolute
  and, apart from the patient's pre-morbid health,
  depend on the site and age of the infarct.
  The important criteria are:
  - ischaemic chest pain of less than 12 hours duration
  - ST elevation in two contiguous leads [or new onset
    left bundle branch block (LBBB)]
  - no unacceptable contraindications.
- Streptokinase is still generally the thrombolytic of
  choice, however t-PA and r-PA are being increasingly
  used—especially for patients under 75 years of age
  with anterior infarcts of less than four hours duration,
  in the repeat use situation, and in patients with
  coronary artery bypass grafting. Reteplase offers the
  advantage of bolus administration, which may save
  time.
- Any or all of the following may be needed:
  - nitrates (sublingual, spray, topical, IV)
  - morphine IV
  - aspirin (used routinely unless allergy is documented)
  - beta-blockers
  - diuretics, inotropes, angiotension converting enzyme
    inhibitors and calcium channel blockers.
- Although not readily available in many centres at
  present, there is clear evidence that acute angioplasty
  is an excellent therapy for reperfusion in acute AMI,

particularly when stenting and platelet inhibitors are used. Its role will increase with availability. It is the treatment of choice in AMI with cardiogenic shock, and should be considered where there are contraindications to thrombolysis.

THROMBOLYSIS PROTOCOLS IN ACUTE MYOCARDIAL INFARCTION

▼ Indication

- Acute myocardial infarction (< 12 hours of pain).
- ECG changes – either new onset LBBB, or ST ↑ in two anatomically contiguous leads.
- Benefits of treatment thought to outweigh risks.
- Use reteplase if the patient has received streptokinase in the past, or in patients less than 75 years of age, with an anterior infarct less than four hours old.

▼ Monitoring

- Continuous ECG.
- Heart rate and blood pressure every five minutes during infusion.

▼ Potential risks

Allergy

- Steptokinase in the past [tissue plasminogen activator (TPA) is preferred]
- Documented strep throat in the last month
- Known allergy to streptokinase.

Bleeding

- Congenital bleeding disorder (e.g. haemophilia)
- Acquired bleeding disorder (e.g. liver disease)

- Recent major trauma (e.g. subdural)
- Recent surgery (e.g. cholecystectomy)
- Medical conditions that may be complicated by bleeding (e.g. haemorrhagic cerebrovasular accident, peptic ulcer)

Note: prolonged CPR and age are not themselves contraindications.

▼ Administration

- Streptokinase: 1.5×10^6 units infused over 60 minutes (note heparin is not required).
- Reteplase: 10 mg IV bolus repeated at 30 minutes (note give heparin 5000 U prior to first dose and then as an infusion at 1000 U per hour after the second dose).

▼ Side effects

- Hypotension, usually only after streptokinase (treated by head tilt down, fluid bolus, stopping then slowly restarting if necessary).
- Haemorrhage.
- Arrhythmias.
- Anaphylaxis.
- Fever, chills, rashes (delayed).

MULTI-TRAUMA

▼ Clinical features

The key to managing multi-trauma in the emergency department is a coordinated, task orientated, team approach. On the medical side, the team is usually:

- a doctor in overall charge (the 'thinker' rather than the 'doer')
- an airway doctor — may also gain central venous line neck IV access
- a procedures doctor, for peripheral IV lines, catheters, etc.

Each doctor in the team should be paired with a nurse. The early involvement of inpatient teams is also needed to ensure rapid movement to definitive care.

▼ Management

The priorities remain the airway, breathing and circulation though, in practice, the team approach allows a number of issues to be dealt with concurrently.

Intubation

Intubation, if needed, requires:

- rapid sequence intubation technique
- cricoid pressure
- sedation with midazolam, fentanyl, or both (thiopentone is potentially dangerous as it causes significant hypotension in the hypovolaemic patient and should not be used by the inexperienced)
- paralysis with suxamethonium to ensure optimal intubating conditions
- tube position confirmed with endotracheal CO_2 monitor before cricoid pressure is released

- maintenance of neck position by in-line stabilisation and not traction

Intravenous fluids

- A young fit patient who is hypotensive on arrival must have lost at least one third of blood volume and, hence, requires blood. Do not delay in commencing blood transfusion in these patients.
- Begin with colloid or crystalloid. After 1500 mL colloid or 3000 mL crystalloid use blood.
- Group specific blood (checked for Rh, ABO) takes much less time to obtain and, in practical terms, causes no more adverse reactions. O-negative is acceptable if time is absolutely critical.

Urinary catheterisation

- Catheterisation is safe in the absence of blood at the meatus, perineal haematoma, high riding prostate on rectal examination, or major pelvic injury.
- If in doubt, perform a urethrogram which can be done quickly and easily in the emergency department.

Investigating the abdomen

- Haemodynamically unstable patients require surgery in theatre and not investigation in the emergency department.
- In general, CT scan is the investigation of choice because of the extra anatomical information obtained, and because it is non-invasive.
- Reserve diagnostic peritoneal lavage for cases where computed tomography (CT) scan or ultrasound is impractical (such as in the mass casualty situation) or unavailable. Diagnostic peritoneal lavage is now only infrequently used in Australasia.

BURNS

▼ Clinical features

Burns may be classified as superficial, partial thickness or full thickness. Superficial burns are typically red, painful, have normal sensation, and blanche on pressure—sunburn is an example. Partial thickness burns are typified by blistering, but sensation remains intact. Full thickness burns are typically grey or white, with little pain, a hard, often leathery texture, and absent sensation.

The rule of 'nines' is used for estimating burn size in adults, with 18% for front and back of the torso, 9% for each arm and 18% each leg, 9% for the head and neck, and 1% for genitals. A useful guide is that the palm of the hand represents 1% body surface area (BSA).

Patients should be admitted with burns of greater than 10% BSA or less if full thickness, and for burns in particularly important areas such as face, hands, feet, perineum or over a major joint. Patients should also be admitted if they have burns which are circumferential, infected or electrical in aetiology.

▼ Management

As with all emergencies, patients with major burns should have immediate attention paid to the airway, breathing and circulation. Don't forget the possibility of carbon monoxide and cyanide poisoning and airway burns. Look for carbonaceous deposits in the nose and throat and singed nasal hairs. Early intubation saves later airway problems in airway burns.

With all burns, rapid cooling of the burn with cold water minimises continuing damage. Protect the burnt area with sterile towels soaked in saline. Do not apply creams or ointments which will need to be removed later. Do not try to remove adherent clothes or hot material, rather cool the area rapidly with water.

An IV cannula should be inserted and generous narcotic analgesia provided as soon as possible. Fluid requirements are large in the first 24 hours and can be estimated with the modified Parkland formula as follows:

Fluid requirements (mL) = BSA × weight × 3 mL.
   in first 24 hours   (%)   (kg)

Give half the fluid in the first 8 hours as normal saline or other electrolyte solution. So for a 20% burn to a 70 kg man, give 2100 mL in the first 8 hours, and 2100 mL over the next 16 hours. Maintenance requirements should be added to this.

Prophylactic antibiotic cover is not used, because it encourages the emergence of resistant strains of organisms.

In circumferential burns, escharotomy may be required.

A variety of dressings has been used for the management of minor burns, including Fixomul, Opsite, paraffin gauze, etc. None seems superior to any other, but all provide protection during healing.

VOLUME RESUSCITATION

It is easy to underestimate a patient's requirements for volume resuscitation in the setting of acute blood loss. The relative efficacy of patients' compensatory mechanisms may mean that the same degree of blood loss will present differently in different patients.

Nevertheless it is possible to estimate blood loss on clinical grounds:

- < 10% circulating blood volume loss leads to little or no signs or symptoms
- 10–20% produces tachycardia and postural hypotension
- 20– 40% produces progressive hypotension (the pulse may slow as the loss nears the upper end of this range)
- > 40% loss is the maximum unreplaced loss that can be sustained.

These effects are magnified in the elderly. Young, fit patients defend their blood pressure with compensatory tachycardia until around a third of blood volume is lost. Elderly patients develop hypotension much sooner and tachycardia is less common.

It is also easy to underestimate blood loss into concealed sites. Some typical losses into various areas include:

- fractured tibia and fibula (750 mL)
- fractured neck of femur (1000–1500 mL)
- fractured shaft of femur (2000 mL)
- fractured pelvis (up to 5000 mL or more).

Which fluid to use depends on the clinical situation and the urgency of the volume resuscitation.

Some points to bear in mind are:

- the crystalloid versus colloid debate is unresolved
- polygeline expands the plasma volume more for the same volume infused, but is expensive
- normal saline is cheap but only 20% of a given volume remains within the vascular space
- 5% dextrose is not a volume resuscitation fluid
- low titre O-negative blood is a scarce resource but is extremely safe and should be used if necessary rather than delaying transfusion
- group specific blood takes only 10 minutes to prepare and carries minimal risk of incompatibility
- fully cross-matched blood may take 30 minutes to obtain.

For volume resuscitation the ideal intravenous access is a pair of short (1 1/4 inch or 3 cm) 14G or 16G cannulae. Larger bore cannulae make little difference to outcome and are difficult to insert. Long cannulae (2 inch, or 5 cm, plus) just slow flow rates. A pressure infusion bag at 300 mmHg maximises IV flow rates. Central venous lines are not indicated for rapid transfusion as their length results in very slow flow rates.

HEAD INJURY

▼ Clinical features

Head injury is a common presentation to the emergency department. The aims of management are to:

- minimise further brain injury in the critically ill patient
- identify those with or at risk of developing a surgically remediable intracranial collection
- provide information and advice to those being discharged home from the emergency department following head injury.

Assessment of the head-injured patient can be difficult and the history often unreliable. A head injury can be assumed if the patient has an altered neurological assessment or if there is a clear history of retrograde amnesia (no memory of the events immediately preceding the head injury). Loss of consciousness can be reasonably assumed if there is no memory of the actual blow to the head. The best widely recognised measure of conscious state is the Glasgow Coma Scale (GCS) which measures best motor, verbal and eye-opening responses as follows:

- Eye opening:
  - spontaneous   4
  - to speech   3
  - to pain   2
  - nil   1
- Verbal response:
  - orientated   5
  - confused   4
  - inappropriate words   3
  - incomprehensible sounds   2
  - nil   1
- Best motor response:
  - obeys commands   6

– localises to pain	5
– withdraws to pain	4
– abnormal flexion	3
– extensor response	2
– nil	1

The maximum score possible is 15 and the minimum 3.

Investigation of a head-injured patient is still a matter of some debate, clouded by the presence or lack of investigational facilities in some centres. The following points can be made.

- Time is a valuable tool, either in the patient with a GCS score of 14 or 15 or those with lower GCS scores who seem to be intoxicated and are improving.
- CT scan is indicated for all patients with GCS scores less than or equal to 13 or those who deteriorate while being observed. An exception may be the intoxicated patient. Some centres with easy access to CT investigate all head-injured patients regardless of GCS score.
- Skull X-rays are generally only indicated for clinically suspected depressed skull fractures. All other patients are better investigated with a CT scan. It is illogical to perform a skull X-ray if CT is planned.

▼ Management

The head-injured patient with GCS score of 8 or less, or one who is deteriorating rapidly, should be managed vigorously. Therapies to consider include:

- rapid neurosurgical referral of any patient with suspected extradural or subdural haematoma
- rapid sequence intubation and hyperventilation to an endotracheal CO_2 of 30–32 mmHg
- nursing with 30 degree head up tilt if possible
- draining the stomach with a nasogastric tube, or orogastric tube if there is any possibility of a fractured base of the skull

- keeping well sedated with morphine/midazolam
- mannitol (0.5–1.0 g/kg IV) if rapidly deteriorating and localising signs
- maintaining cerebral perfusion with a mean arterial pressure of at least 70 mmHg by volume loading if necessary.

CERVICAL SPINE X-RAYS

▼ Clinical features

There is now reasonable agreement about which patients suffering neck trauma warrant X-rays of the cervical spine. Views of the cervical spine are warranted if any of the following criteria apply:

- as part of a 'trauma series' in multi-trauma
- if definite neurological symptoms or signs are present
- if there is midline cervical tenderness
- if the patient has an altered mental state (e.g. head injury/drugs)
- if the patient has a major distracting injury (e.g. multiple rib fractures).

The converse also holds true. If *none* of the above criteria applies then cervical X-rays are not indicated.

If the films are ordered then the patient should be X-rayed lying flat and wearing a hard collar. Allowing a patient to sit up wearing a collar is illogical. Either have the patient lie down or decide the collar is not indicated.

When reviewing cervical spine X-rays use a systematic approach. Remember the lateral is the most important but not the only view. It will show nearly all unstable injuries (> 90%) and most cervical fractures (> 75%). Look for:

- an adequate view (down to C7/T1)—this may necessitate pulling down both arms as the films are taken
- four smooth lines:
  - anterior borders of bodies
  - posterior borders of bodies
  - spinolaminar line
  - tips of spinous processes
- the retropharyngeal space, it should be < 7 mm above C4, and < 20 mm from C5–C7
- the atlantodental interval (distance between dens and the anterior arch of the atlas), it should be 3 mm or less.

SHOULDER DISLOCATIONS

▼ **Clinical features**

The diagnosis of anterior dislocation of the shoulder is usually clear clinically, however radiographs are required in all first dislocations and many recurrent dislocations before reduction can be attempted. Always assess neurovascular function thoroughly on initial examination. The ideal radiograph is the axillary lateral view ('scapular Y view') which makes clear both the presence and direction of the dislocation. Anterior is by far the most common (> 90%). Posterior dislocations are notorious for delays in diagnosis. If severe pain makes an axillary view impossible then a transcapular lateral may be the best view achievable. On this view, the glenoid is located by finding the point where the coracoid, acromion and wing of the scapula meet. The coracoid points anteriorly and this allows the relationship of the humeral head to the glenoid to be deduced.

▼ **Management**

Always provide intravenous narcotic analgesia before the patient goes to X-ray. There are innumerable methods of reducing shoulders. Most have a reported success rate of 70–90%. Some are associated with a higher complication rate and requirement for analgesia but may nevertheless be needed because other methods have failed.

The Milch method described below is well tolerated and is suitable for both anterior and posterior dislocations.

- The patient is supine.
- The operator braces a thumb against the patient's humeral head.
- The arm is gently abducted to an overhead position.
- The arm is then externally rotated with gentle traction.

- The humerus often reduces without a palpable clunk.

The scapular manipulation method is also well tolerated but may be difficult in obese or very muscular patients. This technique is as follows.

- The patient is prone.
- The arm is hanging over the side of the trolley with a sandbag or traction provided by an assistant.
- After 5 minutes the inferior angle of the scapula is pushed medially.

Kocher's method, following, is more effective than other techniques in muscular patients or when the presentation is delayed but is associated with more pain and more frequent injuries to the humeral shaft, neck and labrum.

- The patient is semi-erect.
- The elbow is flexed.
- Caudal traction is applied on the flexed elbow.
- The arm is externally rotated, then adducted across the chest.
- Internally rotate the arm to place the hand on the opposite shoulder.

For performance of these techniques, additional analgesia and relaxation is required. With appropriate precautions, consider the use of:

- nitrous oxide
- intravenous morphine/pethidine/fentanyl in titrated aliquots within the bounds of side-effects
- intravenous midazolam titrated in 1 mg aliquots, ensuring the patient remains conscious. Roving eye movements are a good indication of sufficient sedation for reduction. The patient should still be able to respond verbally.

Post reduction X-rays should always be obtained to confirm enlocation. The patient can be discharged with a broad arm sling. Body bandaging is not required. Orthopaedic follow up should be at about one week.

COLLES FRACTURE

▼ **Clinical features**

Colles fracture is the commonest fracture in the elderly. It is defined as a fracture of the distal radius within 2.5 cm of the wrist joint. The typical deformity in Colles fracture is impaction, dorsal displacement, dorsal tilt, radial displacement and radial tilt of the distal fragment. This presents clinically as the classic 'dinner fork' deformity. The reverse fracture to a Colles fracture is Smith's fracture, where the tilt is ventral rather than dorsal.

Complications of Colles fracture include the early complications of median nerve neurapraxia, and late complications of malunion (common), delayed and non-union (uncommon), Sudeck's atrophy and delayed rupture of the extensor pollicis longus tendon.

▼ **Management**

Colles fracture generally requires closed reduction and immobilisation in plaster of Paris if there is any dorsal angulation of a line drawn along the distal end of the radius in relation to a line along the middle of the radial shaft. Failure to reduce such fractures results in significant functional impairment, although small degrees of dorsal angulation may be accepted in the very elderly with significant other problems or disabilities.

Most emergency departments employ intravenous regional anaesthesia to reduce the fracture, although it can be reduced under brachial plexus block (axillary or interscalene), haematoma block or general anaesthesia.

Prior to reduction, an appropriate plaster of Paris back slab should be prepared. Remember to use wide plaster, at least 15 cm in width, so that the forearm will be nearly encircled with plaster. Reduction is achieved by first disimpacting with traction in the line of the radius, then increasing the deformity to ensure good apposition of the posterior cortices of the radius and distal fragment and, finally, applying firm pressure in an ulnarward and ventral direction to correct the deformity. Following reduction, the radius should come out to length so that the radial styloid is 1–1.5 cm distal to the ulnar styloid. Plaster of Paris should be applied and radiographic views performed to check alignment. A collar and cuff or sling should then be applied depending on patient preference.

Most patients do not require subsequent admission and can be discharged when sensation has returned, although occasionally patients with other problems or difficult domestic circumstances may require overnight admission while social supports are arranged.

INTRAVENOUS CANNULATION

There is no substitute for experience in the insertion of intravenous cannulae and everyone has their own technique.

▼ Tips

- Remember standard precautions!
- Gloves are mandatory in the insertion of any IV cannula in any patient.
- Always dispose of your own sharps.
- Clean up any blood spills.

▼ Site selection

- Antecubital veins are fine in the acute resuscitation setting.
- Veins on the back of the hand, using short cannulae so as not to cross the wrist joint, are preferred for most routine IV lines.
- The cephalic vein in the upper arm is well accepted by patients and provides high flow rates.
- In some patients the only peripheral vein to easily cannulate may be the external jugular.
- Venous cutdowns are largely of historical interest.
- In children younger than 5 years an intraosseous needle may be the most rapid form of access.

▼ Size of cannula

- Use 14G or 16G cannulae for volume resuscitation.
- 20G cannulae are fine for slow IV fluids or drug only administrations.

▼ Local anaesthesia

- All cannulae hurt. Physicians can be remarkably tolerant of other people's pain.
- A small carefully placed intradermal bleb of plain lignocaine (~ 0.2 mL) is almost painless and does not destroy venous landmarks. There is ample literature to indicate that this makes IV insertion almost unnoticeable.

▼ Fixing cannulae in place

- Techniques vary.
- Infection rates are probably comparable with most techniques.
- Transparent dressings such as 'tegaderm' seem to be most convenient.

▼ Cannula insertion

- Try to use a 'one-handed' technique so that the other hand can stabilise the skin.
- Free up the cannula from the stylet before insertion.
- Once a flashback is encountered, immediately flatten out the cannula and advance a few millimetres to keep the bevel of the needle in the vein, and ensure the plastic cannula is in the vein, not just the stylet.
- After this, push the cannula forward off the stylet and not the reverse.
- Attaching a needleless injection site to the cannula reduces the risk of needlestick injuries.
- There is little evidence that self-resheathing cannulae reduce the risk of needlestick injuries. The best protection is to use a cannula with which you are comfortable and familiar.

CENTRAL LINES

Central venous catheterisation is a rapid, relatively simple and—in experienced hands— safe technique for emergency venous access. Central lines are usually not needed in the emergency department particularly for rapid volume replacement and advanced cardiac life support, however they are useful in certain situations.

▼ Indications

- Central venous pressure (CVP) monitoring.
- Transvenous pacing wire access.
- Infusing certain drugs.
- Use for central drug delivery in emergencies is more controversial and rapid volume loading is better achieved with standard large bore peripheral intravenous lines.

▼ Contraindications

- The most important is lack of experience of the operator with the technique.
- Distortion of local anatomy.
- Combativeness of the patient.
- Avoid chest approaches in patients with bleeding diatheses (including anticoagulant therapy), with chest wall deformities, or under two years of age.
- In pneumothorax, the central line should be inserted on the same side.

▼ Catheters

- Catheter-over-needle (limited by length).
- Catheter-through-needle (higher risk of catheter tip embolism and more leakage from the vessel

puncture). The catheter should never be withdrawn through the needle.
- Seldinger guidewire (slower).

Experience should be gained with one standard approach, and one alternative technique should the standard approach fail. Of those listed below, the authors favour the infraclavicular with the internal jugular approach as the alternative, and as the preferred approach in children under two years and for those patients with a bleeding diathesis.

When using a second approach, the ipsilateral side should be chosen so that complications such as pneumothorax occur on one side only. The right side is usually chosen because the pleural dome is lower on that side and the left sided thoracic duct is avoided.

Infraclavicular approach

The patient is supine with the arm adducted. The Trendelenburg position does not influence the calibre of the subclavian vein at the point where it is entered in this approach, although it reduces the risk of air embolism. The needle pierces the skin below the junction of the middle and medial thirds of the clavicle. It is directed towards a point about 1 cm above and 1 cm behind the suprasternal notch. The index finger and thumb of the left hand may be used to guide the direction of the needle by placing the finger in the suprasternal notch and the thumb on the costoclavicular junction prior to insertion of the needle, and aiming immediately above and behind the finger in the line between the two digits. Venous blood usually flows back at a depth of 3–4 cm. The catheter should thread freely.

Internal jugular approach

Three distinct approaches are described—the central, anterior and posterior. Again the operator should be familiar with one.

For the commoner central approach, the patient is in the Trendelenburg position as the internal jugular vein is distensible. Valsalva, or temporarily raising the intrathoracic pressure by squeezing the reservoir bag in the ventilated patient may assist insertion. The triangle formed by the two heads of sternomastoid is identified. The skin is pierced at the apex of the triangle and the needle directed downwards at 30–45 degrees along the border of the clavicular head of sternomastoid towards the ipsilateral nipple. Blood should be withdrawn at a depth of 1–4 cm depending on the proximity of the initial skin piercing to the apex of the triangle. If unsuccessful, the needle should be withdrawn and directed more in line with the sagittal plane, towards the ipsilateral great toe.

External jugular approach

The external jugular vein is usually clearly visible with the patient in the Trendelenburg position. A standard peripheral intravenous cannula can be used with the technique, essentially the same as for peripheral placement. Slightly bending the stylet prior to insertion makes this technique easier. This route can be very useful for emergency intravenous access. By using a J-wire through the lumen of this catheter, or de novo, a true central line can then be placed.

Long line approaches

Although time-consuming, these approaches are very safe with minimal complications and are particularly suitable for the inexperienced or occasional operator. They are usually performed through the antecubital fossa.

▼ General precautions

While connecting all central lines, the hub of the catheter should be occluded with the thumb to lessen the risk of air embolism. After connection, the fluid container should be lowered, with free flow of blood backwards indicating correct placement, and a chest X-ray taken to confirm catheter position and the absence of complications.

▼ Complications

These are reported in 5% of cases and are usually:

- pulmonary complications especially pneumothorax (least likely with long line and jugular vein techniques)
- vascular complications, especially arterial puncture.

Complication rate is inversely proportional to the experience of the operator and in experienced hands central venous line insertion is quite safe.

ARTERIAL PUNCTURE

Even after repeated practice, blood gas sampling may remain a difficult skill to master.

▼ Indications

- Blood gas estimation (acid base status, CO_2/O_2 tensions).
- Electrolyte estimations (many labs can do basic electrolytes on a heparinised arterial specimen).

▼ Technique

- Use a small needle (25G) for radial/brachial, and 23G for femoral.
- Remember to pull back the gas syringe plunger prior to use.
- Position the patient to steady the anticipated puncture site or have an assistant hold the limb.
- Place the tip of the index finger of the non-dominant hand over the artery.
- Roll the finger from side to side to 'feel' the course of the vessel.
- Align the rest of your index finger with the direction of the artery.
- Introduce the needle with the bevel uppermost at a 45 degree angle to the skin. Hold the syringe like a dart between the thumb and index finger of the dominant hand.
- Advance the needle until blood returns and the syringe begins to fill (usually only 0.5 mL is required).
- If the first puncture produces no blood, pull the needle back to (but not out of) the skin and aim a few degrees one way or the other of the original course.
- Once the sample is collected and the needle withdrawn, the puncture site needs firm pressure with a cotton wool swab for five minutes.

INTRAVENOUS ARM BLOCK

▼ Indications

- Intravenous arm blocks are usually used for manipulation of wrist and forearm fractures.
- Occasionally they are used for multiple forearm lacerations or foreign body removal.
- They are not generally suitable for use on the lower limb because of the amount of local anaesthetic required.

▼ Preparation

Patient

- Ideally the patient is fasted for four hours in case of complications which may involve regurgitation, although this is largely a theoretical risk, given the safety of the procedure.
- Use the technique with caution in the under-10-year age group.
- Exclude patients with known allergy, sickle cell disease, vascular disease of affected limb or uncontrolled severe hypertension.
- Informed verbal consent is obtained.
- The patient's weight and systolic blood pressure are recorded.
- The patient is supine.
- Insert a small (22G) IV cannulae in the dorsum of both hands.

Equipment

- Monitoring of ECG and SaO$_2$ is warranted.
- Ready availability of oxygen, suction and bag-mask ventilator is mandatory.
- Inform radiology if the image intensifier is required or if X-rays will be done while the cuff is still inflated.

Drugs

- The only local anaesthetic to use is 0.5% prilocaine.
- All other local anaesthetics are specifically contraindicated.
- Adjuvant drugs such as narcotics, benzodiazepines and nitrous oxide may be required.
- The dose of prilocaine is 3 mg/kg (which equals 0.6 × patient weight in kg, given as millilitres of 0.5% prilocaine—so a 70 kg patient requires 42 mL).

Assistants

- Assistance of one other staff member is mandatory.
- Anaesthesia monitoring and procedure are performed by a different operator.

Technique

- Determine the pressure reading on the cuff being used that is required to occlude the brachial pulse in the affected limb.
- Apply padding around the upper arm then firmly apply and secure the cuff.
- Elevate the limb for at least 60 seconds to exsanguinate, applying brachial artery pressure at the same time.
- Inflate the cuff to 100 mmHg above the previously determined brachial artery occlusion pressure.
- Palpate the brachial pulse to ensure the tourniquet has occluded blood flow.

- Inject slowly the dose of prilocaine that has been previously calculated.
- Remove the IV line through which the prilocaine was injected.
- Observe the patient for signs of toxicity throughout the procedure.
- Do not commence the procedure until anaesthesia is achieved (usually requires 7–10 minutes after the anaesthetic was injected).
- The cuff should not be let down until 20 minutes has elapsed and, ideally, is left on no longer than 40 minutes.
- Details of the anaesthetic are recorded.
- Patients are not discharged from the emergency department until normal finger sensation has returned.

▼ Potential complications

In practice, so long as prilocaine is used these are exceedingly rare.

- If toxic drug levels occur in the systemic circulation this will initially manifest as altered sensorium and agitation. This may progress to seizures which are usually short lived.
- If any sign of toxicity is noted:
  - immediately stop any surgery
  - reinflate or improvise a cuff if deflated
  - administer oxygen
  - lie the patient in the left lateral position
  - control prolonged seizures with benzodiazepines or thiopentone
  - treat cardiac arrest along standard lines.

CONSCIOUS SEDATION

Conscious sedation involves judicious use of sedatives and often narcotics to achieve a state of depressed consciousness which usually later results in significant amnesia, but with preservation of protective reflexes. It is useful for the performance of many procedures in the emergency department.

▼ Indications

- Urgent reduction of joint dislocations or grossly displaced fractures.
- Chest tube insertion.
- Semi-urgent cardioversion.
- Other short painful procedures.

▼ Preparation

Patient

- Exclude drug allergies.
- Ideally the patient is fasted but the urgency of the condition may override this.
- Gain informed verbal consent.
- Site an IV line.
- Provide oxygen by face mask at > 6 L/min.

Equipment

- Continuous monitoring of pulse oximetry is mandatory.
- Monitoring of ECG and blood pressure may be required.
- Equipment for bag-mask ventilation, suction and delivery of high flow oxygen must be immediately available.

Drugs

- Typically a narcotic plus benzodiazepine, with or without nitrous oxide and oxygen (Entonox) are used.
- For painful procedures, start with narcotic (fentanyl, pethidine or morphine) given as small boluses at two minute intervals until the patient is comfortable within the bounds of side effects. Equivalent and suitable starting doses are fentanyl 25 µg, pethidine 25 mg, or morphine 2.5 mg.
- The benzodiazepine of choice is midazolam. Initial dose is 1mg. Subsequent doses at 2 minute intervals of 1–2 mg are titrated to clinical effect. The patient should still be able to respond verbally. Roving eye movements are a good indicator of adequate sedation.
- Nitrous oxide is delivered as 'Entonox' which is 50% nitrous and 50% oxygen delivered by a self-triggering mask.
- Antidotes (naloxone and flumazenil) should be kept in the department but are not required at the bedside. In the unusual event of inadvertent overdose, maintaining oxygenation, airway and ventilation manually are all more important than administering antidotes which should be almost never required.

▼ Discharge

- The patient must always be discharged in the company of a responsible adult.
- Discharge should only occur once the patient is able to conduct a lucid conversation and walk unaided.
- Advise the patient not to drink or operate machinery (including driving) for at least eight hours.

SIMPLE NERVE BLOCKS

A variety of simple nerve blocks are useful in the emergency department. They may facilitate suturing, or performance of procedures such as reduction of fractures or dislocations, as well as wound toilet or debridement.

▼ Femoral nerve block

- Use bupivicaine 0.5% (15 mL in an adult, 1 mL/year of life in a child) drawn up in a 20 mL syringe with a 23G needle.
- Place a finger over the femoral artery, parallel to its course and at the level of the inguinal ligament.
- The femoral nerve will lie one finger's breadth lateral to this. Puncture the skin over the presumed site of the femoral nerve and at right angles to the skin.
- Advance the needle and then aspirate to confirm it is not within a blood vessel.
- Inject one third of the local anaesthetic and come back to (but not out of) the skin.
- Now fan the needle in and out laterally, injecting the remainder of the anaesthetic as you go, being careful to aspirate periodically to ensure the needle is not within a vessel.
- Onset of anaesthesia should be within five minutes.

▼ Ulnar nerve block at the wrist

- This block is useful for the management of fifth finger fractures.
- Use 2–3 mL of 2% plain lignocaine and a 25G needle.
- The needle is introduced vertical to the skin at the level of the wrist and just lateral (radial side) to the flexor carpii ulnaris tendon to a depth of 0.5–1 cm.
- Aspirate to confirm the needle is not in the ulnar artery prior to injection.

▼ Digital ring blocks

- The digital nerves are blocked at the base of the proximal phalanx.
- Always use plain lignocaine (1 % or 2 %) no more than 1–1.5 mL per side.
- Place the hand palm down on a stable surface.
- Approach the nerves through the skin on the dorsal surface of the proximal phalanx at the level where a ring would be worn and aiming for the needle tip to finish a little under the skin on the opposite side of the finger.
- A separate puncture is required for each side of the digit.
- As the nerve splits into two branches, dorsal and palmar, ensure anaesthetic is deposited along the whole length of the needle track as the needle is withdrawn.

SUTURING

▼ **Introduction**

Like intravenous cannulation, suturing is a skill best learnt by supervised experience. Nevertheless some pointers are invaluable.

▼ **Anaesthesia**

The pain of local anaesthetic infiltration can be reduced by:
- buffering: add 1 mL 8.4% $NaHCO_3$ to 10 mL lignocaine 1%
- slow injection
- warming the solution
- infiltrating through the wound edges rather than intact skin
- soaking a pad sitting over the open wound in local anaesthetic prior to infiltration.

▼ **Tips**

Remember standard precautions. The use of goggles as well as gloves and a protective gown should be mandatory for suturing. To adequately irrigate a wound requires at least a 20 mL syringe of normal saline flushed into the wound under pressure.

▼ **Suture selection**

A rough guide to suture material selection is:

- knees, parts of trunk   2/0
- lower limbs   3/0
- hands and forearms, scalp   4/0
- finger tips and parts of face and neck 5/0
- eyelids, ears   6/0

▼ Removal of sutures

A rough guide to time until sutures are removed is:

- face, neck   3–5 days
- scalp   5–7 days
- hand   7 days
- upper limbs   7–10 days
- trunk   10–12 days
- lower limbs   10–12 days

To minimise scarring on areas such as the face, alternate sutures may be removed two days earlier than the remainder.

▼ Alternatives to sutures

Cyanoacrylate glue is only suitable for the face and scalp and must only be used by experienced persons on wounds that appose easily (i.e. on wounds that are not under tension).

Not all wounds require suturing and, indeed, many wounds do better without sutures. Choosing to manage a wound without sutures is not a 'cop out'. Dirty, ragged wounds are often best left open with the patient taking antibiotics. Closing such wounds greatly increases the chances of infection. Wounds with a compromised circulation (such as pre-tibial lacerations) are likely to be made worse by suturing and are best treated by the careful repositioning of the skin and the application of tape closures.

URINARY CATHETER INSERTION

▼ Introduction

Urinary catheter insertion is a simple procedure but has a significant complication rate, particularly related to patient dissatisfaction (due to pain) and urinary tract infection (due to poor aseptic technique). Care should be taken to adequately anaesthetise the urethra prior to the procedure and to use a no-touch technique of insertion.

▼ Indications

- Acute urinary retention.
- Monitoring urine output, usually in the critically ill.
- Providing a means of urinary collection in patients with coma.
- Occasionally for collection of a clean urine specimen in patients unable to void.

▼ Contraindications

- In trauma where urethral injury is suspected (blood at the meatus, scrotal or perineal haematoma, or a high riding prostate on rectal examination). In these cases, a urethrogram should be performed.
- If less invasive methods of urine collection are possible.

▼ Technique

- Gown and glove. Use full aseptic technique.
- Clean the exposed urethra and surrounding area with antiseptic and drape.
- Slowly instill 10 mL of commercial lignocaine jelly into the urethra.

- An appropriate catheter (10Fr for children, 18–24Fr for adults) is inserted with a no-touch technique (using instruments to hold the catheter).
- The catheter should be inserted to the hilt in men before inflating the balloon because the first flow of urine occurs while still in the membranous urethra with at least 3 cm to go before clearing the bladder neck.
- Gradually inflate the balloon with saline, stopping if there is pain or resistance.
- Gently pull the catheter until resistance is felt so that the balloon is at the bladder neck.
- Connect to the drainage system.

▼ Complications

- Urinary tract infection. This is related to the asepsis of the procedure and the duration of the catheter remaining in situ (virtually 100% if greater than 10 days).
- Urethral injury, especially if attempting to insert a urinary catheter in unsuspected urethral trauma.

LUMBAR PUNCTURE

▼ Clinical features

Lumbar puncture (LP) is used as a diagnostic procedure in the emergency evaluation of patients with fever, headache, meningism and altered conscious state. When used appropriately in the emergency department, it is a safe procedure with minimal complications. Patients with signs of raised intracranial pressure, papilloedema, or focal neurological signs should first have a CT scan. However, it should be remembered that CT scanning does not reliably detect raised intracranial pressure.

The presence of uniform blood staining in all three tubes of cerebrospinal fluid (CSF) indicates subarachnoid haemorrhage. The presence of leukocytes indicates central nervous system infection, and bacteria are usually also seen on gram stain. Raised CSF protein is a non-specific indicator of central nervous system inflammation.

▼ Indications

- Suspected meningitis.
- Suspected subarachnoid haemorrhage (CT if available is preferred and detects most haemorrhages, but must be followed by LP if negative).
- Other non-emergency indications.

▼ Contraindications

Patients with signs of raised intracranial pressure, papilloedema, or focal neurological signs should not have LP without a prior CT scan. Other contraindications include local infection and bleeding diatheses. Relative contraindications are lack of cooperation, and deformed local anatomy or previous surgery. Lumbar puncture is not a therapeutic manoeuvre—patients in whom bacterial meningitis is likely clinically require urgent antibiotic therapy before LP.

▼ Technique

The patient should be lying comfortably in the lateral position, conventionally left lateral, although LP can be performed with the patient lying on either side. The knees should be drawn up to the abdomen, to open up the interspinous spaces as much as possible. It is technically easier, with practice, to perform the procedure with the patient sitting up if that can be tolerated, as there is less likelihood of the lumbar puncture needle going lateral to the spinal canal. However this means that pressure cannot be easily measured. For the diagnosis of certain conditions, such as meningitis and subarachnoid haemorrhage, this is not of concern.

The smallest sized LP needle which will not bend during insertion over the required distance is chosen, as the incidence of post-LP headache is directly related to the size of the hole the needle makes in the dura. In adults, this usually means a 22G LP needle although, with the smaller distance required for the needle to travel, this may be as small as a 25G needle in small children. The procedure is carried out under full aseptic conditions, with the operator gowned and gloved, and the patient's skin prepared and draped.

Prior to preparing the skin, landmarks should be identified. A circumferential line around the back from the anterior superior iliac spines should cross the L3/4 interspace. This level, or the one above or below, should be chosen for the procedure as this is below the end of the spinal cord. Positioning is critical if the procedure is performed with the patient lying. The shoulders and hips must be perpendicular to the bed. A pillow between the knees often facilitates this position.

Following local anaesthetic infiltration of the skin and subcutaneous tissues, the needle is inserted perpendicular to the back in the side-to-side plane, and aiming about 15–10 degrees cephalad (towards the umbilicus). With the patient in the left lateral position, the bevel should face upwards to ensure dural fibres are split longitudinally to minimise subsequent CSF leak. In the average adult a 'pop' will sometimes be felt at a depth of around 4–5 cm as the ligamentum flavum is pierced, just prior to penetrating the dura. If the needle strikes bone, it is worth asking the patient on which side the pain was felt—if, as is usually the case, the needle has veered to one side of the spinal column, pain on that side indicates the direction in which the needle should be repositioned.

As the needle is being advanced, the stylet should be periodically withdrawn to check whether there is CSF coming back. Once CSF returns, a manometer should be connected (if a CSF pressure reading is required), and then CSF is collected in three tubes, before removing the needle and applying a sticking plaster.

There is no evidence that rest in bed following LP influences the rate of development of post-LP headache, although this is conventionally done for 8–12 hours.

▼ Complications

Post-LP headache occurs in 5–30%. Infection, and cerebral herniation are very uncommon.

HYPOTHERMIA

▼ Clinical features and management

Hypothermia is graded into mild, moderate, or severe on the basis of a core temperature reading. Rectal temperature is the preferred site for temperature measurement however, in hypothermia, the tympanic is a practical and reliable alternative site.

Mild hypothermia: 32–35°C core temperature

- The patient is typically clumsy, dysarthric and shivering.
- The patient is still capable of generating his/her own heat.
- Treat by putting in dry clothes under blankets in a warm room. Warm oral fluids may be given if the patient is conscious.

Moderate hypothermia: 28–32°C core temperature

- The patient typically has depressed conscious state with bradycardia and hypotension.
- There is progressive loss of the ability to thermoregulate.
- Treat by the same method as for mild hypothermia but add warmed, humidified oxygen at 42°C and a forced warm air blanket (such as the 'Bair Hugger') if available. This will heat patients at 1–2°C per hour. If IV fluids are required then they should be warmed.

Severe hypothermia: less than 28°C core temperature

- The patient is comatose and areflexic, often with dilated pupils.

- Signs of life may be difficult to detect but assume a cardiac output if there is a perfusing rhythm on the ECG monitor.
- Slow atrial fibrillation is very common and requires no specific treatment.
- These patients are at high risk of VF if handled roughly, including instrumentation (gentle intubation is safe).
- Non-arrested cases can be treated as for moderate hypothermia.
- Arrested cases need rewarming by lavage of the left thoracic cavity with large volumes (20 L) of fluids (bladder irrigation fluid is ideal) at 40–42°C or by cardiopulmonary bypass if this is available.
- If in VF/VT then shock once. If there is no success, rewarm before trying again. Bretylium was the drug of choice in this situation but, as from May 1997, it is not commercially available in Australasia. Magnesium may also be effective.

Note space blankets do not have any advantage over conventional blankets in a hospital setting. Remember to check for complications such as electrolyte disturbances including low serum magnesium, infection, coagulopathy, raised amylase and rhabdomyolysis (raised creatine kinase).

Prognosis is, in part, related to the degree of hypothermia but mostly to the associated or underlying problems.

HYPERTHERMIA

▼ Clinical features and management

The two disorders most likely to present to the emergency department are heat exhaustion and heat stroke which, to some extent, represent different parts of a continuum. Neuroleptic malignant syndrome is being increasingly recognised.

Heat exhaustion

- A syndrome of loss of body water and electrolytes with symptoms largely due to volume depletion.
- Temperature is < 39°C and neurological function is intact.
- Treat with rest and oral/IV normal saline/dextrose solutions.

Heat stroke

Features

- A true medical emergency which has a high mortality if treatment is delayed. These patients have lost hypothalamic control of temperature regulation.
- Core temperature is typically > 41°C.
- Neurological dysfunction ranges from coma to hemiplegia.

Treatment

- Vigorous cooling is the key.
- Spray with luke warm water and fan at room temperature.
- Put ice packs in the groin, axillae and on the neck.
- Use minimal IV fluids.
- Control shivering and movement with diazepam or paralysis.

- Aspirin and paracetamol are ineffective.
- Watch for complications such as electrolyte disturbances, pulmonary oedema, disseminated intravascular coagulation, rhabdomyolysis.
- These patients always require management in the intensive care unit after the emergency department.

Neuroleptic malignant syndrome

- This is an idiosyncratic reaction to phenothiazines and sometimes other neuroleptic agents.
- It is characterised by:
  - hyperthermia
  - autonomic instability
  - confusion
  - rigidity.
- Patients may require active cooling and volume resuscitation.
- The treatment of choice is the dopamine agonist bromocriptine.
- Consider referral to the intensive care unit in all cases.

NEAR DROWNING

▼ **Clinical features**

The major pathology is arterial hypoxaemia and the mainstay of treatment is its correction.

Consider co-morbidities in the initial assessment:

- children—child abuse or hypothermia.
- adolescents and adults—alcohol or drugs, hypothermia, cervical spine injury, head injury, epilepsy, arrhythmias or hypoglycaemia.

▼ **Management**

Treatment

- Give 100% oxygen (either bag-mask or via endotracheal tube) initially.
- Have a low threshold for intubation and ventilation (e.g. Glasgow Coma Scale score of 13).
- Positive end expiratory pressure (PEEP) or continuous positive airway pressure (CPAP) may be very helpful.
- Bronchodilators may be necessary.
- Electrolyte and glucose disturbances are rare but should be sought.

Ongoing monitoring

- Close clinical observation.
- Serial arterial blood gases and chest X-rays.

Disposition

- Even apparently minor cases should be observed for 4–6 hours.
- Symptoms, chest signs, hypoxaemia or chest X-ray abnormalities at 6 hours mandate admission.

Prognosis

Children do better than adults. Those conscious or semi-conscious on arrival generally do well but long-term neurological sequelae are common in those comatose on arrival.

AEROMEDICAL TRANSPORT

The essence of aeromedical retrieval is planning and preparation. In general, any problem that may develop or procedure that may be required should be dealt with before takeoff. To predict such events requires an understanding of the pathophysiology of the aeromedical environment.

The major physiological changes at altitude relate to the decreasing atmospheric pressure with increasing height above sea level. This leads to expansion of trapped gas and decreasing inspired partial pressure of oxygen. In addition, the aeromedical environment is noisy, cramped, poorly lit, cold, subject to vibration and motion stress and may have incompatible electrical systems.

The issues with which you need to deal are:

- type of craft
- destination and route planning
- staff
- equipment
- the patient.

Choices in the type of craft, its route and related equipment are, at times, not in the control of the treating medical practitioner. Helicopters are fast and flexible over the 50–200 km range but cannot be pressurised and are particularly subject to excess noise and vibration.

The key issue with staff selection is to choose personnel who are self-reliant and familiar with the aeromedical environment. Whether they are doctors, nurses or paramedics is less important.

For the patient, the key issues are hypoxia and trapped gas expansion. Supplemental oxygen helps both problems. Venting of cavities (for instance, a chest tube in pneumothorax) and pressurisation will be needed to overcome trapped gas expansion. In this regard, medical conditions of particular concern are pneumothorax, open head injury, penetrating eye injury and bowel obstruction.

TOXICOLOGY: COMMON INGESTIONS

▼ Clinical features

Alcohol, benzodiazepines, tricyclic antidepressants and paracetamol are the commonest agents used in self poisoning. These are usually the result of deliberate self harm although, occasionally, may be recreational.

▼ Management

Gastrointestinal decontamination

Charcoal

Activated charcoal is effective against most poisons with the notable exceptions of metals such as lithium, iron and lead. Charcoal is also ineffective in adsorbing alcohol. Corrosive agents (because of the risk of further damage) and hydrocarbons (because of rapid absorption) are also considered contraindications to charcoal. Apart from these exceptions, charcoal is routine therapy in poisoning at a dose of 0.5–1.0 g/kg via nasogastric tube or orally.

Emesis

Emesis with syrup of Ipecac is very rarely used in the hospital setting.

Gastric lavage

Lavage is less frequently used now, except in poisoning that is large, presents early and may delay gastric emptying. The most obvious example is massive tricyclic antidepressant (TCA) poisoning. It may also be used where charcoal is ineffective (such as in lithium poisoning). If performed, meticulous attention to airway protection and proper technique is mandatory.

Most patients who require gastric lavage also require intubation. The Glasgow Coma Scale (see 'Head Injury', page 37) may be an unreliable guide in poisoning to the effectiveness of the gag reflex. Some patients with GCS scores as high as 13 may require intubation for you to safely perform lavage. All patients with GCS scores of 10 or less should be intubated for lavage. If in doubt, it is safer to intubate before lavage rather than risk aspiration. Lavage should be performed through a large bore tube (at least 32Fr). Use warm tap water, approximately 200 mL each time, then empty. Lavage until the effluent is clear (usually about 1500–2000 mL).

Catharsis

Catharsis may cause electrolyte disturbances and is not routinely recommended.

Whole bowel irrigation

This is achieved by administering oral or nasogastric polyethylene glycol solution (such as 'Golytely') at ~ 1000 mL/h until the rectal effluent becomes clear. It may be highly effective in poisoning with slow release preparations, and in iron poisoning.

Specific poisons

Tricyclic antidepressants

Tricyclic antidepressants (TCAs) have a high risk of serious toxicity in overdose. One gram can cause serious morbidity although some TCAs are more toxic than others. There is a high risk of death with 2–4 g. TCAs depress the conscious state initially but the most dangerous effects are broad complex tachyarrhythmias and seizures. The first sign of this serious toxicity is a sinus tachycardia and broadening of the QRS complex on the ECG (due to quinidine-like effects on the heart). At this point, prophylactic administration of 50–100 mL of 8.4%

$NaHCO_3$ over 10 minutes is indicated. Intubated patients should also be hyperventilated to a pH of 7.50. The effect of these two therapies is additive and they act to lower the unbound (and hence toxic) proportion of the drug. Patients with major tricyclic poisoning should be monitored in the emergency department or the intensive care unit and not the coronary care unit because airway problems are common. A patient six hours post-overdose, who manifests no signs of serious toxicity, is unlikely to do so and can be safely considered to be medically clear.

Paracetamol

Paracetamol causes death by delayed liver failure. In adults, 6 g has caused hepatocellular damage and 15 g has caused death. Blood levels taken at four hours post-ingestion are compared to the Rumack nomogram that relates level to time post-ingestion. If the level falls into the 'toxic' range then treatment with IV N-acetylcysteine is commenced. N-acetylcysteine is ideally begun less than 12–15 hours post-ingestion but recent work suggests it may be effective when given up to 24 hours post-ingestion. This delayed approach should always be considered in a patient with massive paracetamol overdose who presents late. The N-acetylcysteine is given by a three-stage IV infusion on the basis of the patient's bodyweight. Allergic reactions are common and may be quite severe but can generally be treated by simply stopping and slowly restarting the infusion. In those rare cases of patients who manifest true anaphylaxis to N-acetylcysteine, an alternative may be high dose IV cimetidine.

Benzodiazepines

Benzodiazepines cause respiratory depression. That alone is not usually a problem if adequate support is provided. They potentiate the effects of other drugs in a polydrug overdose. The specific benzodiazepine antagonist flumazenil may be used to reverse a benzodiazepine overdose, however this is rarely done. Flumazenil can cause seizures in a patient taking a polydrug overdose (especially including TCAs) or habituated to benzodiazepines and frequently causes an unpleasant acute withdrawal reaction with agitation, tremor and tachycardia.

Alcohol

In most cases, supportive care of airway, breathing and circulation is the only treatment required. Alcohol poisoning particularly in the young may lead to quite severe hypoglycaemia and this should be sought for and treated. Patients who are not habituated to the effects of alcohol may need airway and respiratory support at levels as low as 0.25 g/dL.

Narcotics

Narcotic overdose leads to severe respiratory depression. Naloxone (0.4–4 mg) IV or intramuscular (IM) is an effective and safe antidote, however there are some practical problems with its use. It has a duration of action measured in minutes, which is shorter than that of most narcotics so resedation is a real risk and a particular problem if the patient has left the emergency department. Many patients awoken with naloxone given for an accidental 'recreational' overdose become quite aggressive and may insist on leaving the emergency department. For these reasons many emergency physicians prefer to simply support the patient's ventilation and allow the patient to wake up spontaneously.

Antidotes

Specific antidotes may be of value in a limited range of cases. Some of those available include:

- naloxone for narcotics
- N-acetylcysteine for paracetamol

- flumazenil for benzodiazepines
- ethanol for methanol and ethylene glycol
- pyridoxine for isoniazid
- chelating agents for heavy metals
- kelocyanor for cyanide
- fab antibodies for digoxin
- pralidoxime and atropine for organophosphates.

A few drugs that may seem innocent but are particularly lethal and must always be carefully managed are:

- slow release theophyllines
- slow release Ca^{2+} blockers
- beta-blockers
- iron
- isoniazid
- chloroquine
- colchicine
- paraquat.

CARBON MONOXIDE POISONING

▼ Clinical features

Carbon monoxide (CO) is the most common agent used in successful suicide in Australasia. It is a colourless, odourless gas and, hence, often causes accidental poisoning as well, particularly where engines, heaters or cookers are run in confined spaces. Many cases of accidental CO poisoning appear to go undetected.

Suicide by CO poisoning is commonly attempted by victims setting up hoses from the exhaust outlet to the interior of the car, although this is less likely to be fatal now because the introduction of catalytic converters in cars running on unleaded petrol means the CO output is much lower. Patients trapped in burning buildings often develop CO poisoning and this should be specifically examined for in the emergency department. Cyanide toxicity frequently accompanies this situation.

As well as displacing oxygen from haemoglobin, CO is a cellular toxin, directly producing hypoxia at a cellular level. Mild CO poisoning results in non-specific symptoms including headache, nausea, diarrhoea, and cognitive disturbances. With increasing exposure, patients become confused and disorientated, progressing to coma and convulsions. The cardiovascular system may also be affected, with ischaemia, arrhythmias and hypotension. Delayed neuropsychiatric sequelae (extrapyramidal effects, ataxia, impaired higher functions) are common (10–40%) in patients not treated with hyperbaric oxygen (HBO).

Carboxyhaemoglobin (COHb) levels may help to confirm the diagnosis but correlate poorly with clinical outcome.

▼ Management

Initial management, as in all emergencies, involves stabilisation of airway, breathing and circulation. The half life of COHb is dramatically reduced when patients breathe 100% oxygen, and this may need to be supplied by positive pressure ventilation if the patient is comatose or cannot tolerate the 100% mask. There is considerable controversy about the role of HBO in the treatment of CO poisoning, although most authorities would argue it improves outcome.

Currently accepted indications for HBO are any of the following:

- COHb > 25% in the emergency department (15% in children)
- a history of loss of consciousness
- other end-organ ischaemia (for example angina, ECG abnormalities or arrhythmias).

SNAKE ENVENOMATION

▼ Clinical features

Australian snakes are the most venomous in the world, causing profound systemic effects—namely coagulation disturbances, paralysis and myonecrosis, and sometimes renal failure and haemolysis, depending on the snake genus. Most Australian snakes are defensive and will not approach humans unless disturbed.

The diagnosis of snake envenomation is clinical together with the results of investigations. Investigations include coagulation profile (including fibrinogen degradation products or D-Dimer), creatine kinase, and urea and electrolytes. Once envenomation has been diagnosed, antivenom must be given—the sooner the better!

Identify the genus of snake so that the appropriate monovalent antivenom can be administered. This minimises the risk of allergic reactions. Do not attempt visual identification of the snake if it has been brought with the patient. Patients still die because of incorrect snake identification. Use the Snake Venom Detection Kit (VDK) developed by the Commonwealth Serum Laboratories, which enables detection of the genus of snake in many cases, usually from a swab of the wound. The VDK should not be used to diagnose envenomation. If doubt persists about the snake genus, use polyvalent antivenom, which contains antivenom to all major snake genera within a given area. In some regions, where the snake genera are limited, monovalent antivenoms are more appropriate when the snake is unidentified. For instance in Tasmania, tiger snake antivenom covers all snake species in the region; in Victoria, tiger plus brown snake antivenom is sufficient; on Rottnest Island, brown snake antivenom should be used.

Snake antivenoms are derived from horse serum. The rate of allergic reaction is low at less than 5% for polyvalent and 1% for monovalent.

▼ Management

- Apply a pressure-immobilisation bandage if not present.
- Gain IV access, commence cardiac monitoring.
- Adrenaline 0.25 mg may be given intramuscularly (optional).
- Consider giving promethazine (25 mg IV) and hydrocortisone (100 mg IV).
- Give monovalent IV antivenom (polyvalent if uncertain of snake genus*) 15 minutes after adrenaline. Several doses may be needed. Remove the pressure-immobilisation first aid.
- Tetanus prophylaxis should be provided as appropriate.
- To prevent serum sickness, oral steroids (prednisolone 50 mg/day for 5 days) should be given to those receiving polyvalent or multiple doses of monovalent antivenom, and to children in appropriate doses

Important points

- The dose of antivenom should be titrated against response. Many ampoules may be needed.
- The dose is the same for adults and children.
- Skin testing does not predict the occurrence of allergic reactions and should not be performed prior to antivenom administration.

* Note: In Victoria, tiger snake plus brown snake antivenom and, in Tasmania, tiger snake antivenom should be given rather than polyvalent antivenom when the snake has not been identified.

RED-BACK SPIDER ENVENOMATION

▼ Clinical features

The red-back spider is one of the widow spiders, closely related to the American black widow, the South African knoppie and the New Zealand katipo. After an effective bite, the victim develops local pain, erythema and sweating, and sometimes piloerection. Local sweating and piloerection are almost pathognomonic.

About 25% of patients progress over hours to systemic effects, with remote or generalised pain and sweating, vomiting, and nonspecific features such as headache, nausea, hypertension and tremor. If untreated or inadequately treated, this syndrome may persist for up to several months.

Red-back spider antivenom is derived from horse serum. The rate of immediate adverse reactions is 0.5%. There have been no recorded deaths from red-back spider envenomation since the introduction of the antivenom in 1956.

▼ Management

- For patients with mild local symptoms only:
  - give simple analgesics, and review next day
  - admit to the observation ward if worsening
- For patients with severe local symptoms or significant systemic effects:
  - gain IV access
  - commence cardiac monitoring
  - adrenaline (0.25 mg) may be given subcutaneously (optional)
  - red-back spider antivenom 500 units (one ampoule) should be given IM 15 minutes after adrenaline (if used)

- if, after 2 hours, there is incomplete resolution of symptoms, repeat the dose (several doses may be needed)
- intravenous use of the antivenom is only justified when the patient is in extremis (in such cases all patients should be pre-treated with adrenaline, as the incidence of allergic reactions is much higher than following IM administration)
- provide tetanus prophylaxis as appropriate.

BOX JELLYFISH ENVENOMATION

▼ Clinical features

The world's most venomous animal, *Chironex fleckeri*, commonly known as the box jellyfish is found in the warm tropical waters of northern Australia. This large box-shaped jellyfish has caused over 70 deaths in Australia. Typically, an unsuspecting swimmer moves through the long and difficult-to-see tentacles and immediately emerges from the water in considerable pain. The severity of envenomation depends on the extent of contact and the body weight of the victim. Death can occur within minutes—particularly in children.

Locally, affected areas have swollen purple, reddish-brown streaks where the tentacles have contacted the victim. These may ulcerate over days and take many weeks to heal, often leaving permanent scars. The lethal component of the venom affects the heart muscle and respiration. Patients suffer agonising pain, may lose consciousness and have severe cardiovascular disturbances, with shock and tachycardia alternating with hypertension.

Antivenom is derived from sheep serum and has been available in Australia since 1970. It is associated with a very low incidence of allergic reactions and, hence, adrenaline premedication is unnecessary. Antivenom is indicated for continuing pain or difficulty with breathing, swallowing or speaking following adequate first aid. It appears to be effective for other species of box jellyfish as well as *Chironex*.

▼   Management

First aid

- Remove the victim from the water to prevent drowning.
- Pour vinegar over affected areas to inactivate the tentacles.
- Gently remove the tentacles to avoid further venom discharge.
- Commence CPR, if indicated.
- Pressure-immobilisation first aid is controversial. It retards the spread of venom, but may therefore exacerbate local symptoms.

Specific medical management

- Ensure first aid is adequate (further vinegar and tentacle removal may be required).
- Gain IV access.
- Commence cardiac monitoring.
- Dilute the antivenom 1:10 with normal saline.
- One ampoule (20 000 U) is given intravenously for moderate envenomation, but the dose should be titrated against effect and several ampoules may be required.
- Cardiovascular and respiratory support may be required.
- Provide tetanus prophylaxis as appropriate.

STONEFISH ENVENOMATION

▼ Clinical features

Stonefish envenomation causes severe, agonising pain and may be life-threatening. Stonefish are found around the coast of the northern half of Australia. They live in coral reefs or mud flats and their highly effective camouflage makes them look like pieces of rock or coral. They may be nearly impossible to see in the water. The venom glands are on the fish's dorsal spines and cause problems when the fish is stepped on. The victim feels immediate pain which quickly increases in severity. The affected part soon becomes swollen and tender due to local tissue damage, and the victim may develop weakness and paralysis of the affected limb and systemic autonomic features.

Effective antivenom, derived from horse serum, has been available since 1959. Each ampoule contains 2000 U and the initial dose is one ampoule IM per two puncture wounds but, again, antivenom is titrated against effect and more may be needed. In the 12 months to June 1990, 26 patients were treated in Australia with stonefish antivenom, most of them stung on the feet. Eight of the patients required more than one ampoule.

▼ Management

If there is only one puncture wound and mild discomfort:

- clean the wound
- immerse in water as hot as tolerable
- give simple analgesics
- monitor the patient's progress.

If pain is worsening, or for more severe stings, with significant pain or systemic features:

- give antivenom
- gain IV access
- commence cardiac monitoring
- give adrenaline (0.25 mg) subcutaneously (optional)
- give stonefish antivenom 2000 U (one ampoule) IM for every two puncture wounds (several doses may be needed)
- intravenous antivenom may be required in severe envenomation (pretreat with adrenaline)
- wound care may be needed
- provide tetanus prophylaxis as appropriate.

BLUE-RINGED OCTOPUS ENVENOMATION

▼ Clinical features

The blue-ringed octopus is found all around Australia's coastline. It is very small, weighing from 10–100 g, and found in shallow water and rock pools. Although yellowish brown normally, when disturbed, the animal's rings turn brilliant blue. It is the most dangerous of the octopi because of its extremely potent venom, which contains the paralysing neurotoxin tetrodotoxin (identical to that found in the flesh of pufferfish).

The blue-ringed octopus is not aggressive and usually bites only when picked up. The bite is often painless but, within minutes, depending on the amount of venom injected, profound neuromuscular paralysis develops. Death is by respiratory paralysis. The victim, who remains conscious until hypoxia supervenes, can be kept alive with simple expired air resuscitation.

▼ Management

First aid at the scene

- If the victim is conscious, apply pressure-immobilisation first aid and transport rapidly to an emergency department, monitoring breathing and conscious state en route.
- If the victim is unconscious, check for breathing and pulse. If a pulse is present but the patient is not breathing, commence expired air respiration. This continues until definitive artificial ventilation is commenced.
- If pulse and breathing are absent, commence CPR, transport rapidly to an emergency department.

In hospital

- If the victim is conscious, with pressure-immobilisation in place:
  - gain IV access
  - commence cardiac monitoring
  - remove the bandage and observe, being prepared to intubate and ventilate.
- If the victim is unconscious, with pulse present and expired air respiration in progress, perform rapid sequence intubation and ventilation.
- If a pulse is absent, commence standard advanced cardiac life support.

STATUS EPILEPTICUS

▼ **Clinical features**

This is defined as continuous seizures or repeated seizures with failure to regain consciousness in between. If lasting longer than 30 minutes, then severe metabolic disturbances and the potential for serious brain injury ensue.

▼ **Management**

The priorities in management are to:

- maintain oxygenation with 100% oxygen by bag-mask
- exclude hypoglycaemia early by fingerprick estimation
- control fitting:
  - initially diazepam up to 15 mg IV in an adult (give as 5 mg boluses) or midazolam up to 10 mg IV (midazolam can be given IM in a dose of 0.2 mg/kg—this is preferable to rectal diazepam and works just as quickly)
  - clonazepam (1–2 mg IV) may be effective when midazolam or diazepam is not and may be an effective preventative treatment.

Other choices when fitting is not controlled include:

- phenytoin (15 mg/kg IV over 30 minutes)
- phenobarbitone (15 mg/kg over 15 minutes)
- thiopentone with which doctors may be more familiar
- $MgSO_4$ (5g IV over 5 minutes).

Once fitting is controlled a loading dose of phenytoin is usually given, as above, if this has not already been done.

When to intubate in status epilepticus is a difficult question. Paralysis does not stop cerebral seizure activity and fitting must also be controlled.

Consider diagnoses other than primary epilepsy when prolonged seizure activity is encountered. Possible aetiologies include:

- poisoning (salicylates, TCAs, theophylline, amphetamines)
- cerebral infections
- metabolic disturbances (hyponatraemia)
- cerebral mass lesions or haemorrhage
- heat stroke.

MIGRAINE

▼ Clinical features

Whether a headache is a true migraine or mixed tension/vascular headache is probably irrelevant in terms of emergency department management. What is important is that other more serious diagnoses (in particular subarachnoid haemorrhage and meningitis) have been excluded by history, examination and, if needed, investigation (lumbar puncture, CT scan).

▼ Management

A number of drug therapies are likely to be effective in up to 90% of patients. All cases should be rested in a quiet, darkened room. Drug choices include:

- metoclopramide (10 mg IV) followed 15 minutes later by paracetamol (1500 mg) or aspirin (900 mg orally)
- prochlorperazine (12.5 mg IV slowly)
- chlorpromazine (12.5–37.5 mg IV in 12.5 mg increments every 20 minutes)
- sumatriptan (6 mg subcutaneously)
- dihydroergotamine (1 mg IV).

Because of their low cost, ready availability, efficacy and low recurrence rate the first three of the above drugs are probably preferable. Any of these drugs can cause dystonic reactions and sedation. Prochlorperazine and chlorpromazine can cause postural hypotension, and patients should be pretreated with a bolus of 500 mL of normal saline intravenously.

The use of pethidine for migraines is strongly discouraged. Apart from its obvious addiction potential it is no more effective than other therapies (and may be less so) and has by far the highest headache recurrence rate.

SUBARACHNOID HAEMORRHAGE

▼ Clinical features

Subarachnoid haemorrhage (SAH) should be considered in the differential diagnosis of any headache because it is life-threatening and may present quite subtly. Although the diagnosis is often thought of when patients present moribund after sudden collapse, patients may be quite well, with no signs but simply complaining of headache. Clues to the diagnosis are the sudden onset of severe headache, the 'worst ever' headache, and headache in patients who never get headaches. Symptoms and signs of meningism may or may not be present.

Patients are graded according to the Hunt and Hess classification as shown in the table below.

Grade	Signs
(i)	Alert, with or without meningism
(ii)	Drowsy with no neurological signs
(iii)	Drowsy with neurological signs
(iv)	Deteriorating with major neurological deficit
(v)	Moribund with failing vital centres

Complications

Complications include rebleeding in 16–25% of patients with a peak incidence at day 4–9, and vasospasm, which occurs in 40–70% of patients and is responsible for most of the morbidity and mortality.

Investigation

The question of whether CT should precede lumbar puncture is controversial. CT does not reliably detect raised intracranial pressure. In the absence of ready availability of CT, it appears that LP is safe as a first investigation if the patient has a normal conscious state and no focal neurological signs. If CT is performed first, an LP is mandatory to exclude the diagnosis of SAH if the CT is normal.

▼ Management

Comatose patients should be managed with general supportive care as usual. Care should be taken with rapid sequence intubation to ensure reflex rises in intracranial pressure are minimised. This can be achieved by using high dose fentanyl (2–3 µg/kg) with induction or pretreatment with lignocaine 1.5 mg/kg three minutes prior to intubation, although the evidence that these agents prevent such rises is limited.

Hypertension should be controlled with sedation, analgesia and antihypertensives. Drugs such as beta-blockers and hydrallazine are preferred to vasodilators which may produce cerebral vasodilation and raised intracranial pressure. Calcium channel blockers such as nimodipine have been shown to improve outcome. Some authorities recommend phenytoin loading to reduce the risk of seizures which result in raised intracranial pressure.

Grade (i) to (iii) patients are usually operated on early, with postoperative hypervolaemic haemodilution to minimise the risk of vasospasm.

Recognition of small 'warning' subarachnoid haemorrhage is vital, as Grades (i) to (iii) when identified and treated early generally have a good prognosis. Untreated, further catastrophic bleeding is likely.

COMA

▼ Clinical features

Coma may be the end result of a variety of clinical conditions. It is defined as depression of cerebral responsiveness. A useful way of assessing level of cerebral responsiveness is the Glasgow Coma Scale (see 'Head Injury', page 37). It is generally accepted that a GCS score of 8 or less equates with coma. Causes may be categorised as intracranial and extracranial.

Intracranial

Causes include:
- vascular events, such as stroke
- infection
- neoplasm
- seizures
- injury.

Extracranial

Causes may be:
- toxic
- metabolic
- endocrine
- infective
- cardiovascular .

Investigations are directed at finding the cause and will be guided by clinical findings. The priorities are ensuring oxygenation and excluding hypoglycaemia.

▼ Management

The 'coma cocktail' of years gone by (naloxone, glucose and thiamine) is not used now and is potentially harmful.

If narcotics are the cause of coma, assisted respiration is required. If the patient is given naloxone and wakes up and leaves the department against advice, the short half life of naloxone leaves the patient at risk of redeveloping respiratory depression and coma in an unsafe environment. Glucose may exacerbate brain injury after stroke. With rapid fingerprick blood glucose testing, the requirement for glucose can be determined very quickly.

Once a patient becomes comatose, if lying flat on the back, loss of muscle tone enables gravity to cause the tongue to fall backwards and occlude the airway. So early airway control is vital in all comatose patients. Because protective airway reflexes are lost, a cuffed endotracheal tube is the safest method of airway control and protection against aspiration of stomach contents. Ventilation may also be required depending on the cause of coma.

CROUP/EPIGLOTTITIS/ BRONCHIOLITIS

Except in the child who presents truly in extremis or apnoeic, there should be little clinical confusion between these conditions.

▼ Croup

Clinical features

Presents typically at 6 months to 6 years of age with a barking cough, inspiratory stridor and preceding upper respiratory tract infection. In severe cases there may be marked retraction, stridor which may be expiratory as well, and agitation due to hypoxia (confirmed by SaO_2).

Management

Treat severe cases with:
- nebulised adrenaline (5 mL of 1:1000 in a nebuliser bowl)
- parenteral steroid (e.g. dexamethasone, 0.6 mg/kg IM/IV)
- supplemental oxygen if frankly hypoxaemic
- early referral to a paediatric intensive care unit.

▼ Epiglottitis

Clinical features

These children are typically one to four years of age, but the disease is now less common with haemophilus vaccination. It follows a rapidly progressive course.

Children look toxic, cough is absent, and they often sit up with the neck protruded, drooling.

Management

Treat with:
- a gentle, minimum intervention approach
- rapid transport to theatre for gaseous induction anaesthesia and intubation
- bag-mask ventilation until help arrives if the child presented with frank airway obstruction. Intubation with a smaller than usual endotracheal tube may be life-saving in this situation.

▼ Bronchiolitis

Clinical features

These children are usually 3–12 months of age, and present with a respiratory illness and poor feeding. They may have audible wheeze or only grunting respirations and tachypnoea. If severe, they are hypoxaemic ($SaO_2 < 92\%$).

Management

- Nebulised salbutamol can be tried but is rarely effective.
- More severe cases (failure to feed or hypoxaemia) need admission.
- Ventilatory support is not usually required in the emergency department.

CHILD AT RISK (NON-ACCIDENTAL INJURY)

▼ Clinical features and management

Clinical suspicion of non-accidental injury (NAI) mandates instituting a management plan to protect the potentially at risk child from further trauma. In many areas this involves compulsory notification to the responsible authority. In most cases of an emergency department presentation, this requires admission to hospital.

Suspect this condition when the injuries are inconsistent with the stated mechanism, presentation is delayed, or the child is brought to the emergency department by other than the usual care giver. NAI occurs in all social classes.

▼ Common patterns of injury

Soft tissue

- Bruising of varying ages on unusual sites such as upper arms, cheeks, buttocks or perineum.
- Bite marks from adult dentition.
- Burns from cigarette butts or in a hot water dunking pattern.

Bones

- Multiple fractures (such as ribs) at various stages of healing.
- Metaphyseal chip fractures (considered pathognomonic).
- Spiral fractures of long bones in children under two years old.

- Skull fractures with apparently minor trauma.

Shaken baby syndrome

- Bilateral subdurals.
- Retinal haemorrhages.

General

- Severe napkin dermatitis.
- Other signs of obvious physical or mental neglect.

THE FEBRILE CHILD

▼ **Clinical features**

The aims in assessment and management of the febrile child are:

- to initiate immediate therapy for life threatening illness such as septicaemia or seizures
- to perform an appropriate clinical and diagnostic workup to exclude serious infection (pneumonia, meningitis, urinary tract infection)
- to ensure the patient is discharged from the emergency department to the right destination, whether that be inpatient care or home (a necessary part of this being to ensure adequate follow up).

A significant fever is usually defined as over 38.5°C by rectal reading. Children over three years of age rarely present a diagnostic dilemma, as the child may be able to give a history and is more likely to localise symptoms and signs. Younger children can be considered in three groups:

- less than three months of age
- 3–12 months of age
- 12–36 months of age.

At less than three months of age, the safest management plan for the febrile child is a full septic work up and admission.

Between three months and three years, the first step is always a thorough physical examination. If an obvious focus is found, this can be treated. In the child without an obvious focus, the management plan will be influenced by the presumed aetiology, the degree of toxicity on physical examination, the child's age and the availability of community support and follow up. If the white cell count is above 15×10^9/L, then serious bacterial infection is more likely.

▼ Management

Management options include:

- clinical review only at 24 hours (this is inadequate under 12 months or if the review appointment is unlikely to be kept)
- blood cultures and review at 24 hours
- blood cultures, urine specimen (bladder tap or catheter) plus chest X-ray (if there are signs of respiratory illness) then review at 24 hours
- the above plan with the addition of a lumbar puncture (this is especially applicable in the under 12 months group) and review at 24 hours
- any of the above investigative regimens with commencement of empiric antibiotic therapy and then review at 24 hours. Choice of antibiotics includes:
  - procaine penicillin, 1.0×10^6 units IM
  - ceftriaxone, 250 mg IM
  - amoxycillin orally is controversial and may not cover a wide enough bacterial spectrum.

If menigococcal septicaemia or meningitis is suspected clinically, then do not delay treatment awaiting pathology results. Immediately after blood cultures are taken, give empiric therapy with a third generation cephalosporin.

Febrile convulsions are usually short-lived and require no specific initial intervention. More prolonged seizures are usually controlled with midazolam (0.1 mg/kg IV or 0.2 mg/kg IM) or diazepam (0.1 mg/kg IV or 0.2 mg/kg per rectum). Both can be repeated as needed. Hypoglycaemia must be corrected. More prolonged seizures may require phenytoin (15 mg/kg IV over 30 minutes) or general anaesthesia. Cooling measures such as paracetamol (15–20 mg/kg per rectum) and tepid sponging should be commenced but will not terminate an acute seizure.

INTRAOSSEOUS INFUSIONS

▼ **Introduction**

Intraosseous (IO) infusions are indicated for emergency vascular access in the critically ill child less than five years of age, when peripheral venous access (including the external jugulars) cannot be obtained.

▼ **Technique**

- The preferred site is the proximal tibia, two finger breadths below the tibial tuberosity on the anteromedial surface.
- The distal tibia, distal femur, iliac crests and sternum can be used.
- Use a specifically designed IO needle, if possible.
- Direct the needle away from the epiphysis.
- Introduce the needle with a rotary motion.
- A loss of resistance is felt on entering the medulla and position can be confirmed by aspirating blood or fat.

Most conventional IV fluids (including blood) can be infused through such a device. Flow rates can be markedly increased by the use of a pressure bag that is inflated to 300 mmHg. Such a system can achieve a flow rate of 1000 mL in five minutes.

Drugs can be administered in standard IV doses, although clear pharmacokinetic data are lacking. Most conventional resuscitation drugs have been delivered by the intraosseous route. The two drugs contraindicated by this route are $NaHCO_3$ and calcium. Cross match and biochemistry can be performed on blood from a marrow aspirate.

DIABETIC EMERGENCIES

▼ Clinical features

Diabetics may present to the emergency department with an altered conscious state or coma due to either hypoglycaemia or hyperglycaemia. In the emergency department, unlike in the community, the first step is to check the blood sugar with a fingerprick specimen. It is not usually necessary to give intravenous glucose until this result is available (usually 90 seconds).

▼ Management

Hypoglycaemia

Hypoglycaemia manifests classically either as a comatose or a sweaty, combative and confused patient. Treatment is restoration of normal blood glucose with 0.5–1 mL/kg of 50% dextrose intravenously. Elderly patients, in particular, may not wake up 'at the end of the needle' despite a normal blood glucose. Following IV dextrose, the patient should be fed and observed until blood glucose is definitely stable.

Hyperglycaemia

Hyperglycaemia presents as varying degrees of altered conscious state and dehydration. The essentials in early management are:

- rapid restoration of intravascular volume depletion with polygeline or normal saline
- gentle restoration of total body water depletion, initially with normal saline
- a careful search for a precipitating cause (chest X-ray, ECG, urine culture, creatine kinase, amylase)

- careful monitoring of electrolyte disturbances, especially K^+, Na^+, Mg^{2+} and PO_4^{2-} and arterial blood gases
- gentle lowering of blood glucose by insulin infusion (usually ~2–5 units/hour)
- early K^+ supplementation, especially once insulin is started
- careful monitoring of fluid balance. This requires a urinary catheter.

Hyperosmolar coma is treated in a similar fashion to hyperglycaemia. Careful, slow restoration of normal metabolic function and parameters is the key.

ACUTE ANAPHYLAXIS

▼ Clinical features

Anaphylaxis has a broad range of presentations, from a rash to full cardiorespiratory arrest. Patients may present de novo from the community or be affected by drugs administered in the emergency department. Precipitants are varied and frequently cannot be identified. Often, in the emergency department, the precipitant is of little clinical relevance. Antibiotics are the most commonly identified cause. Don't agonise over the cause—immediate treatment is essential.

The systems most commonly affected are skin, lungs, cardiovascular system and gastrointestinal tract.

▼ Management

Mild reactions

- There is usually patchy skin involvement only.
- Treat with oral or IM antihistamines.

Moderate reactions

- These consist of generalised skin reactions and/or bronchospasm and/or mild oropharyngeal swelling.
- Treat with IM antihistamines (such as promethazine, 0.5 mg/kg).
- Salbutamol nebulisers and subcutaneous adrenaline (0.25 mg in an adult) may be required.

Severe reactions

- These consist of a moderate reaction plus hypotension, cardiovascular collapse, or major upper airway obstruction.

- Treat with:
  - oxygen/IV fluids
  - IM adrenaline (0.5 mg in adults)
  - careful IV adrenaline (0.02–0.05 mg/dose) if very sick
  - IM/IV antihistamine
  - IV steroids

Delayed recurrence should be anticipated. All patients with moderate to severe reactions, even if treated and fully resolved, should be observed for a least six hours prior to discharge.

ACUTE PAIN MANAGEMENT

No one modality of pain relief is universally effective or universally applicable. Many options are available in the emergency department.

▼ Entonox

- This consists of 50% oxygen and 50% nitrous oxide.
- It is rapidly effective with a quick offset.
- Entonox is ideal for early pain relief in isolated limb injuries.
- It is excellent as an adjunct to painful procedures such as IV cannulation and suturing in children.

▼ NSAIDs, paracetamol

- These are generally only for mild to moderate pain.
- Rapid acting, non-steroidal, anti-inflammatory drugs (NSAIDs) such as naproxen, diclofenac, indomethacin or piroxicam given per rectum are highly effective in renal colic (though with a slower onset than narcotics).

▼ Metoclopramide, prochlorperazine, chlorpromazine

These are specific treatments for migraine and are more effective than narcotics.

▼ Narcotics

- Should be given as IV aliquots (pethidine 25 mg, morphine 2.5 mg, fentanyl 25 µg) if rapid pain relief is required.

- The right dose is that dose which relieves the pain ('the right dose is *enough*')
- Given judiciously, narcotics do not cloud surgical assessment of the abdomen, and with easy availability of CT can be given without concern in head injury.

▼ Local anaesthetics

- These are often forgotten and underused.
- Can provide better analgesia than any modality in some situations, such as:
  - fractured shaft of femur (femoral nerve block)
  - digital injuries (digital nerve block)

▼ Non-pharmacological methods

Splinting, ice and elevation may also effectively relieve pain.

EPISTAXIS

▼ Clinical features

Epistaxis can occur in many degrees of severity. The main aspects of care are to:

- identify and treat the bleeding site
- recognise and manage hypovolaemia
- consider and manage contributory medical problems.

▼ Management

Emergency department management may consist of some or all of the following.

First aid

- Calm and reassure the patient, ensuring comfortable posture.
- Apply firm pressure on the anterior nares for at least five minutes.

Volume resuscitation

This is dictated by assessed blood loss.

Sedation and analgesia

This is usually achieved with 2.5 mg aliquots of morphine, and often relieves pain-induced hypertension which may be contributing to bleeding.

Topical vasoconstrictors and local anaesthetics

- 2–4% lignocaine with adrenaline may be used.
- An alternative is 4–10% cocaine (use particular caution in the elderly or those with ischaemic heart disease).

- Both of the above are usually applied using cotton wool pledglets.

Anterior nasal packing

- Layered Bismuth iodoform paraffin paste (BIPP) ribbon gauze is packed into the anaesthetised nasal cavity.
- An expanding nasal tampon may be used as an alternative (this needs to be lubricated with KY jelly prior to insertion and may require injection of normal saline to expand).

Posterior nasal packing

- Patients requiring posterior nasal packing should be admitted.
- Use a longer expanding nasal tampon (10 cm) or a Foley catheter.
- Try a purpose-made balloon catheter, such as the Brighton epistaxis balloon.

Cautery

- Cauterise with $AgNO_3$, or by electrocautery.
- This has the potential to worsen the bleeding.

Correction of coagulopathy

This is usually done with fresh frozen plasma for those on warfarin or with liver disease (need to measure the international normalised ratio beforehand).

SUICIDE RISK ASSESSMENT

▼ Clinical features

The screening of potentially suicidal patients aims to identify those at moderate to high risk of self harm and to channel them into a treatment programme. A number of factors when taken in combination can be helpful in such screening.

A useful mnemonic is the 'SAD PERSONS index' which identifies a number of high risk variables:

- S = sex (males are at higher risk)
- A = age (those over 40 years are more at risk)
- D = depression
- P = previous attempts
- E = ethanol
- R = rationality (or lack of, e.g. psychotic patients)
- S = spouse (lack of a partner or significant other)
- O = organised plan of suicide
- N = no supports (no back-up in the community)
- S = sickness (those with chronic illness are at higher risk)

Another useful concept is that of risk/rescue ratios. A high-risk suicide attempt is one where the chosen method has a high expected lethality and a low chance of discovery (low risk of rescue). An example would be driving into a remote forest with a loaded shotgun.

▼ Management

In the emergency department, these patients require:

- emotional support in a non-judgemental manner
- observation, always in sight of staff
- a safe environment without access to potential weapons

- pharmacological intervention if the patient is particularly agitated or disturbed
- referral to a crisis team or acute psychiatric service.

TRIAGE

▼ **Background**

Triage is the process of sorting patients into categories that stratify their urgency for medical assessment. As such, it is the principle that dictates the priority of care provided to all patients presenting to the emergency department.

The National Triage Scale developed by the Australasian College for Emergency Medicine divides patients into one of five triage categories. This is based on a brief and directed nursing assessment conducted at a single triage point at the entrance to the department.

▼ **Definitions**

The categories in the following table are assigned in response to the statement, 'This patient should wait for medical care no longer than ...'

Time interval	National triage category	Number	Colour
'immediately'	Resuscitation	1	Red
'10 minutes'	Emergency	2	Yellow
'half an hour'	Urgent	3	Green
'one hour'	Semi-urgent	4	Blue
'two hours'	Non-urgent	5	White

To aid in identifying the triage categories of patients a coloured dot according to the code above may be applied to the history and the history placed on a coloured clipboard. The box for patients waiting to be seen may be similarly coded, as may departmental computer systems.

Patients should be seen by medical staff in order of their triage category and not on the basis of their arrival time. 'Fast tracking' is not a triage role. If patients are to be seen out of triage order because of local considerations, this is not a triage issue.

Description of the categories

Category 1: Resuscitation, seen immediately

This applies to patients in extremis who would probably suffer significant morbidity or mortality if not attended to immediately. It would include patients with conditions such as cardiac arrest, or airway obstruction, drowning, coma, and so on, where immediate support to airway, breathing or circulation is required to prevent cardiac arrest.

Category 2: Emergency, seen within 10 minutes

This applies to patients with major illness or injury where there is a significant threat to life or limb. This might apply to patients with such conditions as acute severe asthma, myocardial infarction, multiple trauma, significant poisoning or envenomation, chemical burns to eyes, acute abdomen, and so on. Even if the diagnosis is not immediately known, the urgency may be identified by clinical features such as abnormalities in vital signs or high-risk aspects of the history.

Category 3: Urgent, seen within 30 minutes

This category is for patients with possible threats to life or limb, or significant pain requiring rapid relief, such as those with fractures of long bones, renal colic, dyspnoea, abdominal pain, vaginal bleeding, acute psychiatric disorders, and so on.

Category 4: Semi-urgent, seen within 60 minutes

This category is for patients who are suffering some illness or injury which requires medical attention more quickly than could be obtained through an appointment with a general practitioner. This might include conditions such as minor fractures, sprains, soft tissue injuries, minor burns, simple urinary tract infections, a foreign body in throat or eye, minor lacerations, wound infections, minor headache, and so on.

Category 5, Non-urgent, seen within 120 minutes

This refers to all other patients—that is those patients who
are not incapacitated and have no risk to life or limb. Most
could wait for appointments to be seen. This might include
patients with old injuries, any chronic complaint, anxiety,
rashes, attendance for dressings or results, and so on. This
category should not, however, be equated with general
practice or 'inappropriate' attendances.

STANDARD PRECAUTIONS

Emergency departments are high-risk environments for body fluid exposure. The best defence against such exposure is the doctor's own behaviour. The major principles of standard precautions are to:

- regard all patients as potentially infective
- always wear gloves when likely to be exposed to body fluids
- wear gowns, goggles and masks in appropriate situations
- don't recap needles
- always dispose of your own sharps
- ensure your Hepatitis B immunisation is current.

In the event of body fluid exposure:

- wash the area immediately, if appropriate
- always report the episode immediately.

Always follow the department's needlestick/body fluid exposure protocol.

CLINICAL PROBLEMS FOR STUDENTS

The problems on the following pages are designed to highlight important points in some of the major topics covered in this book. It is recommended that you work your way through them with a small group of your colleagues. The information is presented as shown in the following legend.

▼ Legend

i This indicates 'information'. A limited amount of information regarding the problem is given each time.

? This indicates a question aimed at setting you thinking about the given information. (Consider your answer before turning the page each time.)

A This represents a brief answer reflecting the content of relevant sections of the text.

At the end of each problem an outcome is given.

The scenarios evolve in sometimes less than predictable ways but the authors hope you will grant them the 'artistic licence' to do this so that a number of topics can be covered. Remember that, sometimes, despite our best possible efforts, some of our patients die.

PROBLEM 1

ℹ A 21-year-old man, with a known history of schizophrenia, is brought to the emergency department by his friends. They have found him collapsed at home surrounded by a number of empty containers of pills. They believe he took the tablets at least four hours ago.

? What will be your initial brief assessment?

Consider your answer.
Then turn the page.

Initial assessment reveals:

- Glasgow Coma Scale score 7—eyes 2, motor 4, verbal 1
- blood pressure 95/70
- temperature 36.5°C
- pulse 110
- respiratory rate 12
- chest auscultation—right-sided crackles
- pupils—mid-sized and sluggish
- dry skin
- 'poor' gag reflex
- normal skin colour but SaO_2 is 95%
- no external signs of trauma.

Now continue...

i Having completed your initial brief assessment, you must undertake some early definitive management.

? What will be your major priorities in initial management?

Consider your answer. Then turn the page.

Initial management must include:

- intubation (by rapid sequence technique) and ventilation
- intravenous access and volume loading with N saline
- gastric decontamination by aspiration of gastric contents without formal gastric lavage (instillation of activated charcoal)
- early check of fingerprick glucose
- introduction of a urinary catheter.

Now continue...

i The patient is now intubated and ventilated with IV access established and running. Activated charcoal has been given. Observations are:

- blood pressure 105/70
- pulse 120
- SaO_2 99%
- endotracheal CO_2 42 mmHg (5.8 kpa)

? At this stage, what investigations are needed?

Consider your answer.
Then turn the page.

Tests performed should include:

- fingerprick glucose (if not already performed)
- electrolytes
- serum
  - ethanol
  - paracetamol, at more than four hours post-ingestion
  - salicylate
- electrocardiograph
- chest X-ray
- possibly full blood examination, clotting profile, arterial blood gases.

Now continue...

The resuscitation nurse calls you back to the patient. His blood pressure has dropped to 90/60 and pulse to 80. The ECG you ordered is now available and reproduced as Figure 3 below.

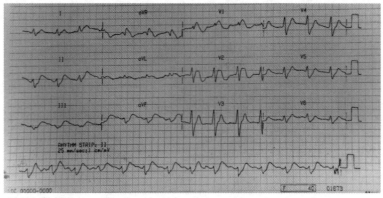

Figure 3

What does the ECG show?

Consider your answer.
Then turn the page.

The ECG shows gross QRS widening and QT prolongation.

Now continue...

i While you are considering the ECG the patient commences to fit. He is still intubated and ventilated.

? Which drug do you think is the one most likely to be causing these effects and what will now be your management?

Consider your answer.
Then turn the page.

The likely diagnosis is TCA poisoning, although any drug with a quinidine-like effect on the heart could possibly cause fitting and these ECG changes.

The priorities now are:

- hyperventilation to a pCO_2 of 30 mmHg (4 kpa)
- 50 mL 8.4% $NaHCO_3$ intravenously over 5 minutes
- seizure control with diazepam.

Now continue...

i The patient is once again stable. Seizures have ceased. Pulse is 90 in sinus rhythm with normal QRS morphology. Blood pressure is 120/80. The serum paracetamol, salicylate and ethanol levels are now available. They are:

- salicylate 0
- ethanol 68 mmol/L
- paracetamol 650 µg/mL

? On the basis of these results, what further action will you now undertake?

Consider your answer. Then turn the page.

The priority is now specific therapy for the paracetamol poisoning with N-acetylcysteine given as a three-stage infusion based on body weight.

Now continue...

i The N-acetylcysteine has now been commenced and the first stage of the infusion run through. The patient develops a generalised blotchy red rash and seems more difficult to ventilate.

? What does this set of findings represent and what action if any will you take?

Consider your answer.
Then turn the page.

The reaction is an allergy/anaphylaxis to the N-acetylcysteine. This is quite common, occurring to a lesser or greater degree in about 15% of patients so treated. In general, the infusion can be continued at a lower rate. Only the most severe reactions require cessation of the infusion and giving subcutaneous adrenaline. In those cases where N-acetylcysteine cannot be continued then high dose IV cimetidine has been suggested as an alternative.

WITH YOUR VIGOROUS TREATMENT THE PATIENT STABILISES AND IS TRANSFERRED TO THE INTENSIVE CARE UNIT.

PROBLEM 2

A 69-year-old woman with a long-standing history of asthma is brought to the emergency department. She complains of two hours of increasing shortness of breath not relieved by her usual puffers at home. She has previously been on inhaled steroids but stopped taking them a few months ago 'because they didn't work'. She has no known allergies. Brief auscultation reveals widespread expiratory wheeze. You make a working diagnosis of asthma.

What initial assessment at the bedside will you undertake?

Consider your answer.
Then turn the page.

The initial assessment is aimed at:

(i) confirming diagnosis (with asthma this is often clear cut)

(ii) assessing severity (see table):

	Mild	Moderate	Severe
PEFR	> 75%	25–75%	< 25% predicted
SaO_2	normal	92–95%	< 92%
Speech	normal	phrases	words or nil
Mental state	normal	normal	increasingly confused

(iii) Looking for complications/precipitants:
- pneumothorax
- pneumomediastinum
- infection
- theophylline toxicity
- long-term steroid use
- hypokalaemia
- arrhythmias.

Now continue...

i Your initial assessment reveals that the patient can talk lucidly, but only in short phrases, her peak expiratory flow rate is 180 L/min and her SaO_2 is 92 % on air.

? What treatment will you now give?

Consider your answer.
Then turn the page.

Treatment for presumed asthma in the emergency
department usually includes:

- non-drug
  - sit up
  - calm and reassure
- drug
  - frequent nebulised salbutamol (5 mg at 30 minute
    intervals)
  - oxygen (including oxygen to drive nebulisers)
  - nebulised ipratropium (0.5 mg up to two-hourly)
  - steroids (she may be well enough to swallow
    prednisolone 1 mg/kg; an alternative is
    dexamethasone, 8 mg IV, or hydrocortisone,
    200 mg IV).

Now continue...

Despite your initial treatment, the patient seems to be making no improvement. She is afebrile. You decide to do a chest X-ray which is reproduced as Figure 4 below.

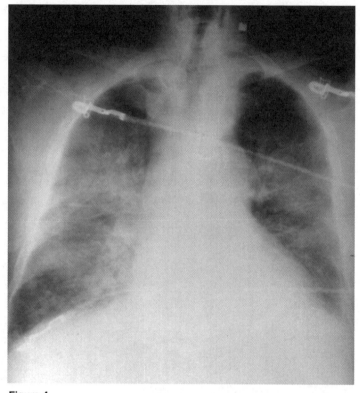

Figure 4

What does the X-ray show?
What will now be your treatment?

Consider your answer.
Then turn the page.

A The chest X-ray shows marked pulmonary oedema. Knowing what the X-ray shows, it is clear that the patient's initial presentation was one of so called 'cardiac asthma'. Typically, pulmonary oedema is due to heart failure but can occur in other settings, such as being drug induced (e.g. heroin, naloxone), or when a pneumothorax is re-expanded, or with anaphylaxis or septicaemia. Treatment typically includes:

- high flow oxygen
- diuretics (e.g. frusemide, 40 mg IV)
- morphine in 2.5 mg IV aliquots
- nitrates sublingually, topically or IV, titrated against blood pressure
- CPAP (probably a good choice here despite possible concerns about barotrauma).

Now continue...

The patient continues to worsen despite vigorous treatment for her pulmonary oedema. She seems to be tiring rapidly and blood gas shows a pCO_2 of 75 mmHg (10 kPa). You decide to intubate to provide peak end expiratory pressure and ventilatory support. Ten minutes after intubation she becomes cyanosed, her pulse increases to 135 and she becomes difficult to ventilate.

What are the likely causes of this rapid deterioration and what is the treatment for each?

Consider your answer.
Then turn the page.

The diagnosis that must be urgently excluded in this scenario is a tension pneumothorax.

- Confirm clinically or on chest X-ray (but only if this is immediately available).
- Treat initially with needle aspiration.
- Later the patient will need tube thoracostomy.

If fulminant pulmonary oedema is the diagnosis then management consists of more of your initial therapy together with intravenous glyceryl trinitrate, inotropes and salbutamol.

Now continue...

A radiographer is immediately at hand, so you ask for a chest X-ray which is reproduced as Figure 5 below.

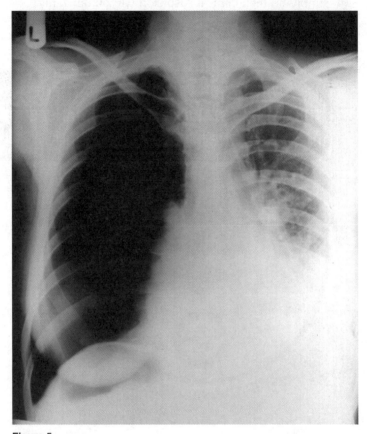

Figure 5

What will you now do?

Consider your answer.
Then turn the page.

An urgent needle aspiration is the most rapid way of treating a tension pneumthorax and can be initiated simply on high clinical suspicion without an X-ray. However, this should routinely be followed with an intercostal catheter.

> **WITH YOUR VIGOROUS TREATMENT THE PATIENT STABILISES AND IS TRANSFERRED TO THE INTENSIVE CARE UNIT.**

PROBLEM 3

You are the medical officer on duty in the emergency department. One of the local general practitioners rings you for advice. She has a 62-year-old male patient with her who has left-sided chest pain and she is querying the possibility of a pulmonary embolism as a diagnosis. You advise her to send the patient by ambulance to you but, while still on the phone, she asks you what is the typical presentation of a pulmonary embolism.

What advice will you give regarding the typical presentation of a pulmonary embolus?

Consider your answer.
Then turn the page.

The diagnosis is not always clear and the onset may be insidious. Many other diseases have features consistent with pulmonary embolism.

- History
  - at risk groups
  - dyspnoea in > 90%
  - chest pain in 50%
  - collapse may occur.
- Examination is rarely helpful except in the massive pulmonary embolism with shock and elevated jugular venous pressure.
- Investigation:
  - hypoxia or increased A-a gradient in most cases
  - ECG changes in > 90% but usually only tachycardia or non-specific ST/T changes (the classic pattern of S_1, Q_3, T_3 is rare)
  - chest X-ray will rarely show a Hampton's hump or Westermark's sign
  - V/Q scan is helpful when a high probability result occurs in a high clinical probability patient (similarly, when low probability scans occur in low clinical probability patients but intermediate results are unhelpful)
  - less than 50% will have signs and test results consistent with a lower limb deep vein thrombosis.

Now continue...

i The patient that you discussed with the general practitioner has now arrived in the emergency department. He looks pale and somewhat clammy. Blood pressure is 150/90. Pulse is 90. Examination of his heart and lungs is normal and his jugular venous pressure is not raised. He is still complaining of chest pain and looks considerably more unwell than you thought he would.

? What will be your plan of management over the next 10 minutes?

Consider your answer. Then turn the page.

Management is based on the assumption that chest pain is cardiac in origin until proven otherwise. Treatment may include:

- monitoring
  - in a resuscitation area
  - continuous ECG
  - non-invasive blood pressure
  - SaO_2
- supportive
  - comfortable posture (usually sitting)
  - oxygen
- drugs (assuming that a cardiac aetiology is likely)
  - aspirin
  - glyceryl trinitrate (spray or sublingual)
  - intravenous morphine in 2.5 mg aliquots
  - intravenous metoclopramide 10 mg
- early investigation
  - ECG is by far the most important
  - K^+ may be indicated
  - group and hold if thrombolysis is considered
  - cardiac enzymes do not help at this stage.

Now continue...

The patient's pain and distress are somewhat relieved by your initial treatment and his observations have remained unchanged. You now have the opportunity to review his ECG which has just been taken. This ECG is reproduced as Figure 6 below.

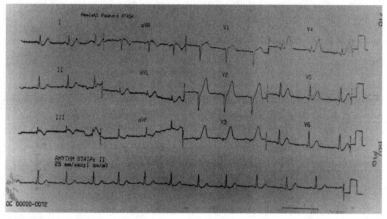

Figure 6

What does this ECG show?
What management will you undertake over the next 30 minutes?

Consider your answer.
Then turn the page.

The ECG shows peaking of the T-waves anteriorly and some ST/T changes inferiorly, suggesting a hyperacute anterior infarct. The management plan should consist of:

- continuation of the measures previously undertaken as necessary
- commencement of a glyceryl trinitrate infusion of 5 µg/min up to 20 µg/min
- ECG repeated in 15 minutes
- immediate consideration of referral to angiography facilities if your hospital has them readily available.

Now continue...

As requested, the patient was commenced on a glyceryl trinitrate infusion. He is now pain free and, in fact, feels much improved though a little drowsy from the morphine he was given. His repeat ECG in 15 minutes is shown to you and is reproduced as Figure 7 below.

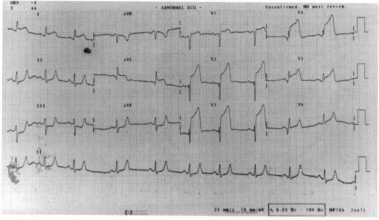

Figure 7

What does the ECG show and what now will be your therapeutic plan?

Consider your answer. Then turn the page.

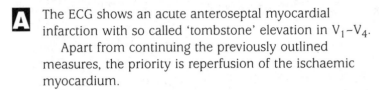

The ECG shows an acute anteroseptal myocardial infarction with so called 'tombstone' elevation in V_1–V_4.

Apart from continuing the previously outlined measures, the priority is reperfusion of the ischaemic myocardium.

- Arguably the best option in this setting is acute angioplasty but this depends on immediate availability of facilities.
- Thrombolysis is the next option and should be given in the emergency department immediately if no major contraindications exist, such as allergy or bleeding diathesis.
  - With an anterior AMI such as this, the benefits of thrombolysis usually outweigh the risks
  - tPA and rPA are most commonly used in this situation, with rPA potentially faster because it is given by bolus rather than infusion. Streptokinase is a cheaper alternative, and may be equally effective.

Now continue...

ℹ Your hospital only stocks streptokinase and there is some available in the emergency department.

? Describe the contraindication checklist to the use of streptokinase, how it is given and common problems encountered when it is used.

Consider your answer.
Then turn the page.

For any patient, there is a risk/benefit analysis, essentially of the risks of treatment against the risks of the disease. Risks from streptokinase are classified as:

- Allergy
  - streptokinase administered more than five days ago (risk of allergic reaction or drug being neutralised by antibodies)
  - known true streptokinase allergy
  - documented strep throat in the past month
- Bleeding
  - congenital bleeding disorder (e.g. haemophilia)
  - acquired bleeding disorder (e.g. liver failure)
  - conditions likely to be complicated by bleeding, such as major trauma, recent surgery or medical disorders (e.g. peptic ulcer, cerebrovascular accident).

Given as an IV infusion of 1.5×10^6 units over 60 minutes with continuous ECG monitoring and 5-minutely blood pressure checks.

Problems
- Hypotension (often 10–15 minutes into infusion) usually responds to lying flat, slowing/ceasing infusion, and volume loading (e.g. polygeline 200 mL bolus).
- Arrhythmias (may be due to 'reperfusion' of ischaemic myocardium).

THE PATIENT IS SUCCESSFULLY TRANSFERRED TO THE CORONARY CARE UNIT POST STREPTOKINASE.

PROBLEM 4

ℹ As the medical officer on duty in the emergency department, you are given advance notification by the ambulance service of the impending arrival of a motorcyclist who has been involved in a high-speed road traffic crash. The only details available are that he is about 20 years of age and is suffering from 'multi-trauma'.

? What preparation will you make before his arrival?

Consider your answer.
Then turn the page.

Preparations would include:

- assembling a resuscitation or trauma team, typically compromised of three pairs of doctors/nurses:
  - one in overall charge
  - one to manage the airway and any procedures in the neck area
  - one to perform all other procedures such as IV access, catheters, chest tubes, etc. and to order pathology and radiology
- ensuring equipment is at hand for:
  - definitive airway control
  - rapid volume infusion (primed IV lines)
  - patient monitoring
- notifying in advance:
  - radiology
  - blood bank
  - operating theatres.

Now continue...

i The patient arrives in the resuscitation room. Handover from the ambulance gives his Glasgow Coma Scale score as 14, pulse 105 and blood pressure 100/60 all of which are confirmed by the nurse who takes the initial emergency department observations.

? By the end of the first 10 minutes, what goals do you consider the team should have achieved?

Consider your answer.
Then turn the page.

The goals should be:

- gaining control of airway, breathing and circulation (from the little history so far available it is likely these are reasonably stable)
- instituting volume resuscitation (just the patient's observations and the mechanism of injury suggest that he has significant blood loss—typically the fluid would be given through two 16G or larger cannulae placed in the antecubital fossae)
- completing a head-to-toe examination to elucidate what injuries are likely clinically—key points often neglected are:
  - checking the ears for blood and/or cerebrospinal fluid
  - a gross neurological screen
  - checking the urethral meatus for blood
  - rectal examination
- protecting the cervical spine initially with a hard collar
- providing appropriate initial analgesia.

Now continue...

By the end of 10 minutes, the patient's observations are essentially unchanged. He has been given nearly one litre of Haemaccel intravenously. Your examination finds no sign of significant head or spinal trauma, tenderness over his left 9th, 10th, and 11th ribs laterally, diffuse lower abdominal tenderness, pain on springing the pelvis and a deformed right thigh.

What injuries do you consider likely?
What analgesia will you provide?
What investigations would you perform?

Consider your answer.
Then turn the page.

The likely injuries on the basis of the clinical details so far are:

- fractured left lower ribs
- suspected splenic injury
- fractured pelvis
- minor head injury
- fractured right shaft of femur.

Analgesia could consist of:

- aliquots of morphine, 2.5 mg at a time, given with 10 mg of metoclopramide initially (there is no reason to withhold morphine even if a head injury is present)
- a femoral nerve block with 15 mL of 0.5% plain bupivicaine (this is likely to be effective, minimise the need for narcotics and allow a traction splint to be applied)
- Entonox, which may be a useful initial adjunct but there are possible concerns regarding associated chest injury

Investigations must include:

- cervical spine views
- chest X-ray
- pelvis X-ray
- cross match blood (ask for two units, group specific)
- a urethrogram, depending on clinical findings
- serum ethanol.

Now continue...

The patient's observations still remain unchanged, but you now have available his basic trauma radiology. His lateral cervical spine seems normal and the chest X-ray shows a fractured left 10th rib.

What do the X-rays of his pelvis and femur (reproduced below as Figures 8 and 9) show?

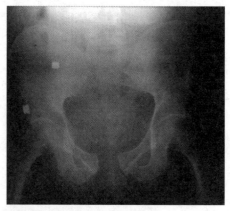

Figure 8: Pelvis X-ray.

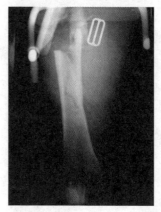

Figure 9: Femur X-ray.

Consider your answer.
Then turn the page.

The pelvis X-ray shows diastasis of the symphysis pubis and fractured sacrum.

The femur X-ray shows a comminuted, displaced angulated fracture of the right femoral shaft.

Now continue...

The patient now has a Glasgow Coma Scale score of 15. Pulse and blood pressure have changed little with blood pressure currently 105/70 and pulse 100. He has received 1000 mL of Haemaccel, 1000 mL of N-saline and has two bags of group specific blood running.

What further investigation is now required?

Consider your answer. Then turn the page.

The investigation that is now required is still a matter for some debate, though most clinicians would favour the first of the following approaches:

- CT scan of the abdomen/pelvis with gastrointestinal contrast will provide the most anatomical information with the highest sensitivity—but is more costly, time consuming and cannot be done in the resuscitation room.
- Diagnostic peritoneal lavage can be performed easily in resus but is less sensitive and doesn't provide anatomical information. Frank blood when the needle is inserted is an indication for immediate laparotomy.
- Urethrogram.
- Ultrasound is used by some centres for assessing abdomens in multi-trauma to identify free intraperitoneal fluid.

Now continue...

i You choose to take the patient for CT scanning. Just after he is lifted onto the CT slide, his pulse is 130, his blood pressure is 70 systolic and he is becoming increasingly confused.

? What will you do now?

Consider your answer.
Then turn the page.

Actions required now are:

- to notify theatre, anaesthesia, general surgery and orthopaedics that the patient is en route to theatre
- to increase volume resuscitation to maximum rates
- to order six more units of group specific blood urgently
- to apply a military anti-shock trousers suit, in particular the pelvic compartments, on the assumption that the major source of bleeding is pelvic, and in an attempt to reduce the potential space
- pelvic fixation and laparotomy.

AFTER A STORMY COURSE IN THEATRE AND THE INTENSIVE CARE UNIT, THE PATIENT EVENTUALLY SURVIVES.

PROBLEM 5

You are at the beach in late autumn. A speed boat comes racing to shore with a body slumped in the back. Knowing you are a doctor, the locals urgently call you over. The patient is a 49-year-old local fisherman whose small boat has capsized out in the bay. He was found floating in the water wearing a buoyancy vest. They picked him up only a minute ago but have not been able to gain any response since. He feels cold to touch, has a pulse of 90 but looks cyanosed and does not appear to be breathing. Just how long he has been immersed is not clear as his companion has not yet been found.

What initial steps will you take?

Consider your answer.
Then turn the page.

The priorities in this situation are:

- airway and breathing—mouth-to-mouth, mouth to mask, bag-mask, endotracheal tube—use whatever method is available
- to prevent ongoing heat loss and protect from wind, e.g. with a space blanket, cutting off the patient's wet clothes and using dry blankets
- to protect his cervical spine with a hard collar, if possible
- to deliver oxygen at the highest flow rate possible
- urgent transfer to an emergency department.

Now continue...

You accompany the patient in the ambulance to the emergency department. With initial mouth-to-mouth and, later, bag-mask ventilation he has begun to breath himself. On arrival in the emergency department his pulse is 60, blood pressure 90/50, respiratory rate 12, Glasgow Coma Scale score 8 and temperature 34°C by rectal reading.

From what conditions might he be suffering?
What initial investigations are needed in the emergency department?

Consider your answer.
Then turn the page.

The likely diagnoses, and those that need to be considered, include:

- near drowning
- hypothermia
- trauma
  - cervical spine injury
  - head injury
- medical conditions causing loss of consciousness
  - sub arachnoid haemorrhage
  - seizures
  - acute myocardial infarction/cardiac arrhythmia
  - drug ingestion (especially alcohol)
  - dysbarism
  - envenomation.

Investigations required include:

- chest X-ray, cervical spine X-ray
- ECG
- blood gas
- urea and electrolytes, Mg^{2+}
- glucose
- full blood examination
- clotting profile
- serum ethanol.

Now continue...

The investigations have now been performed. The blood gas shows relative hypoxaemia but all other biochemistry and haematology are normal. The chest X-ray shows patchy right upper zone opacification. There is no reason to believe the diagnosis is other than hypothermia and near drowning. The patient's ECG is reproduced as Figure 10 below.

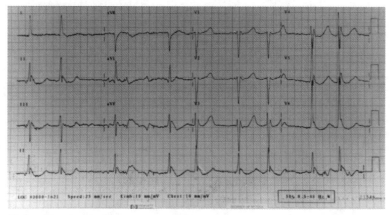

Figure 10

What does the ECG in Figure 10 show?
What management will you undertake in the emergency department?

Consider your answer.
Then turn the page.

The ECG shows slow atrial fibrillation and J waves consistent with hypothermia. Management priorities are:

- hypothermia—at 34°C the patient should be able to passively rewarm himself by being placed in a warm, dry, wind-free environment, e.g. gown and multiple blankets (any IV fluids given should be warmed)
- near drowning—the key is correction of hypoxia (this patient should be intubated and ventilated—careful watch needs to be kept for progressive hypoxaemia, onset of pulmonary oedema, coagulopathy and renal injury).

Now continue...

The intubation is a particularly difficult one because of the patient's receding jaw and bull neck. You succeed in placing the tube but, as you do so, the ECG monitor shows the patient has gone into VF. Surprised that this should occur at this temperature, you note that the thermometer used for the temperature readings is a standard glass model. You ask for an immediate tympanic temperature, which is 28.4°C. CPR has been commenced.

How will you now manage this scenario?

Consider your answer. Then turn the page.

Management should include :

- continued ventilation via endotracheal tube
- single 200 J DC shock
- if successful, commencement of rewarming using humidified oxygen and a forced air rewarming blanket.
- if no response
  - continued CPR
  - urgent rewarming using left thoracic lavage or cardiopulmonary bypass
  - trying reshocking at 29°C, 30°C, 31°C, 32°C as the patient rewarms
  - cessation of efforts if the patient is 32°C and still in VF.

> **DESPITE ACTIVE REWARMING, THE PATIENT REMAINED IN VF AND RESUSCITATION WAS DISCONTINUED.**

PROBLEM 6

A 58-year-old man is brought to the emergency department by ambulance. He has a past history of a cardiomyopathy which is thought to be ischaemic or alcoholic. Over the past three days he has had frequent 'dizzy spells and funny turns'. Today he collapsed at the returned serviceman's club and his friends called the ambulance. He is conscious and alert, somewhat intoxicated but quite cooperative. His blood pressure is 100/60, pulse 60, respiratory rate 16 and he is afebrile. He has been put on a monitor in the resuscitation room. As you arrive, the resus nurse hands you his ECG which is reproduced as Figure 11 below.

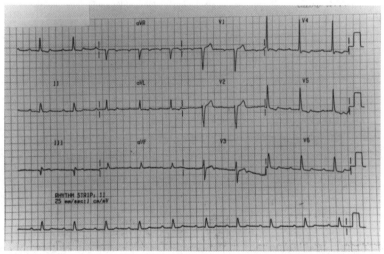

Figure 11

What does the ECG show?
What will be your initial investigation and management plan?

Consider your answer.
Then turn the page.

The ECG shows:

- first degree heart block, rate 60 beats per minute
- lateral ischaemia

Management should consist of:

- continuous ECG monitoring
- oxygen
- checking of electrolytes especially Mg^{2+} and K^+
- cardiac enzymes
- serum or breath alcohol
- full blood examination
- chest X-ray
- plans to admit for continuous ECG monitoring.

Now continue...

i You go to organise the patient a bed in the low acuity area in the coronary care unit. The resus nurse says the patient has developed a tachycardia and looks somewhat pale and clammy but his blood pressure remains 100/60. You ask for another ECG to be performed. This ECG is shown as Figure 12 below.

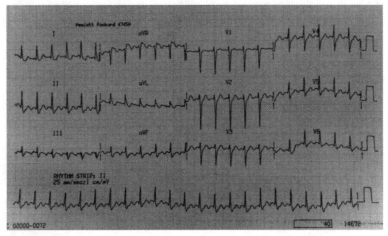

Figure 12

? What does the new ECG show?
How will you now treat him?

Consider your answer.
Then turn the page.

The ECG shows:

- a regular narrow complex tachycardia at 150 beats per minute [this could be paroxysmal supraventricular tachycardia (PSVT) or atrial flutter with a 2:1 block]
- there is widespread but minor ST segment depression.

Treatment should consist of:

- continuous ECG, O_2 (already in place)
- trying vagal techniques (e.g. Valsalva) to either 'unmask' atrial flutter or possibly to revert PSVT
- adenosine, only if vagal measures fail and PSVT is suspected (6 mg via antecubital vein as a rapid IV push, followed by 12 mg two minutes later if required)
- sedation with midazolam then cardiovert with 25–100 J synchronous DC shock, if adenosine fails or atrial flutter is suspected.

Now continue...

■ The second dose of adenosine successfully reverts the patient. Initially he goes into sinus rhythm but he then goes into a new brady arrhythmia. Again he looks pale and clammy and blood pressure is 90/60. Another ECG is performed and is shown as Figure 13 below.

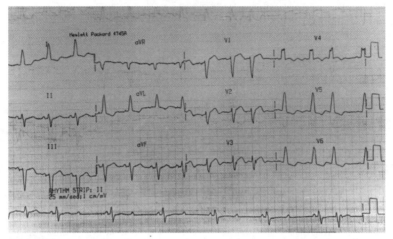

Figure 13

❓ What does the ECG show?
How will you now manage the patient?

**Consider your answer.
Then turn the page.**

The ECG shows:

- bradycardia, ventricular rate approximately 40 and second degree atrio-ventricular block on the rhythm strip
- sinus rhythm with LBBB on the rest of the ECG.

The key points in management other than the other issues already covered are:

- to apply a trans-cutaneous pacemaker now as a precautionary and therapeutic measure
- make arrangements for urgent insertion of a transvenous pacemaker.

Now continue...

The patient deteriorates further. He is now only semi-conscious with palpable femoral pulses but no recordable blood pressure. The resus nurse is fetching the trans-cutaneous pacemaker while another ECG has just been done. This EGC is shown as Figure 14 below.

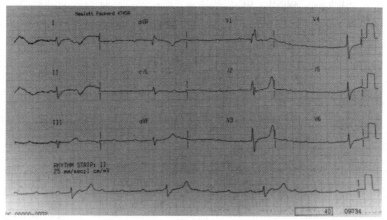

Figure 14

What does the ECG show?
How will you manage the patient now?

Consider your answer.
Then turn the page.

The ECG shows:

- complete heart block
- ventricular rate of approximately 20
- atrial rate of approximately 100.

The management is:

- ideally to apply and operate the trans-cutaneous pacemaker now
- atropine (up to 1.2 mg IV may be given as a temporising measure)
- dopamine/isoprenaline infusions are at best second line therapies
- transvenous pacing, which can be commenced when practical.

Now continue...

ℹ The patient is now stable with the trans-cutaneous pacer
functioning, although he required IV midazolam to tolerate
it. You choose, nevertheless, to insert a transvenous pacing
wire. As you advance the wire into the right ventricle his
rhythm again changes. He still has clearly palpable
brachial pulses but his conscious state is hard to gauge
because of the midazolam. Another ECG is taken and is
shown as Figure 15 below.

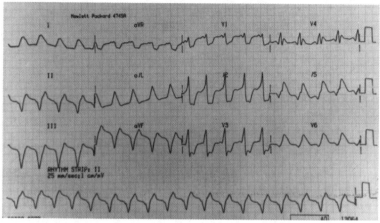

Figure 15

❓ What does the ECG now show?
How will you manage this rhythm?

Consider your answer.
Then turn the page.

The ECG shows:

- broad complex tachycardia at 150 beats per minute
- no evidence of fusion or capture beats
- what is very likely to be ventricular tachycardia, especially given the clinical scenario.

Management is:

- to pull back the pacing wire
- lignocaine (1.5 mg/kg IV)
- cardioversion, as a consideration if lignocaine fails
- $MgSO_4$ (2.47 g IV) may be very useful especially in this patient who is likely to be hypomagnesaemic.

Now continue...

Despite the lignocaine, the patient deteriorates further. There are now no pulses palpable. His respiration has ceased. His monitor rhythm strip is shown as Figure 16 below.

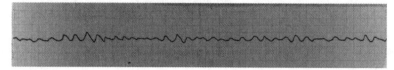

Figure 16

What does the monitor rhythm strip show?
How will you manage this rhythm?

Consider your answer.
Then turn the page.

A The rhythm strip shows ventricular fibrillation.
The management is:

- to commence a full advanced cardiac life support protocol
- for a witnessed arrest, defibrillate first with
  - 200 J
  - 200 J
  - 360 J
- adrenaline (1 mg IV given every 3–5 minutes)
- intubation early in arrest, then 100% oxygen
- to repeat 360 J DC shock 60 seconds after every drug given
- consideration of second line drugs, including
  - lignocaine
  - $MgSO_4$
  - KCl
  - $NaHCO_3$

DESPITE YOUR FULL RESUSCITATION ATTEMPTS, THE PATIENT DIED.